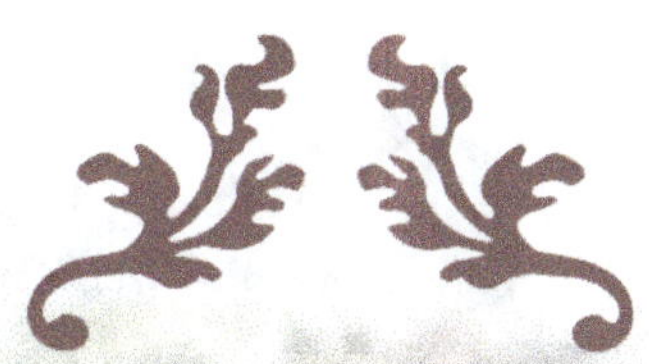

THE GALVESTON DIET COOKBOOK 2024

Easy and Delicious Recipes with Nutritional Values and Health Benefits for a Vibrant Life

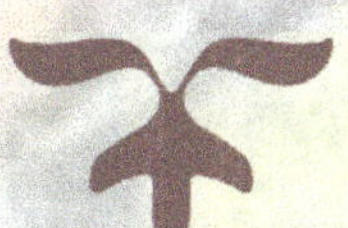

JOEY RAMSEY

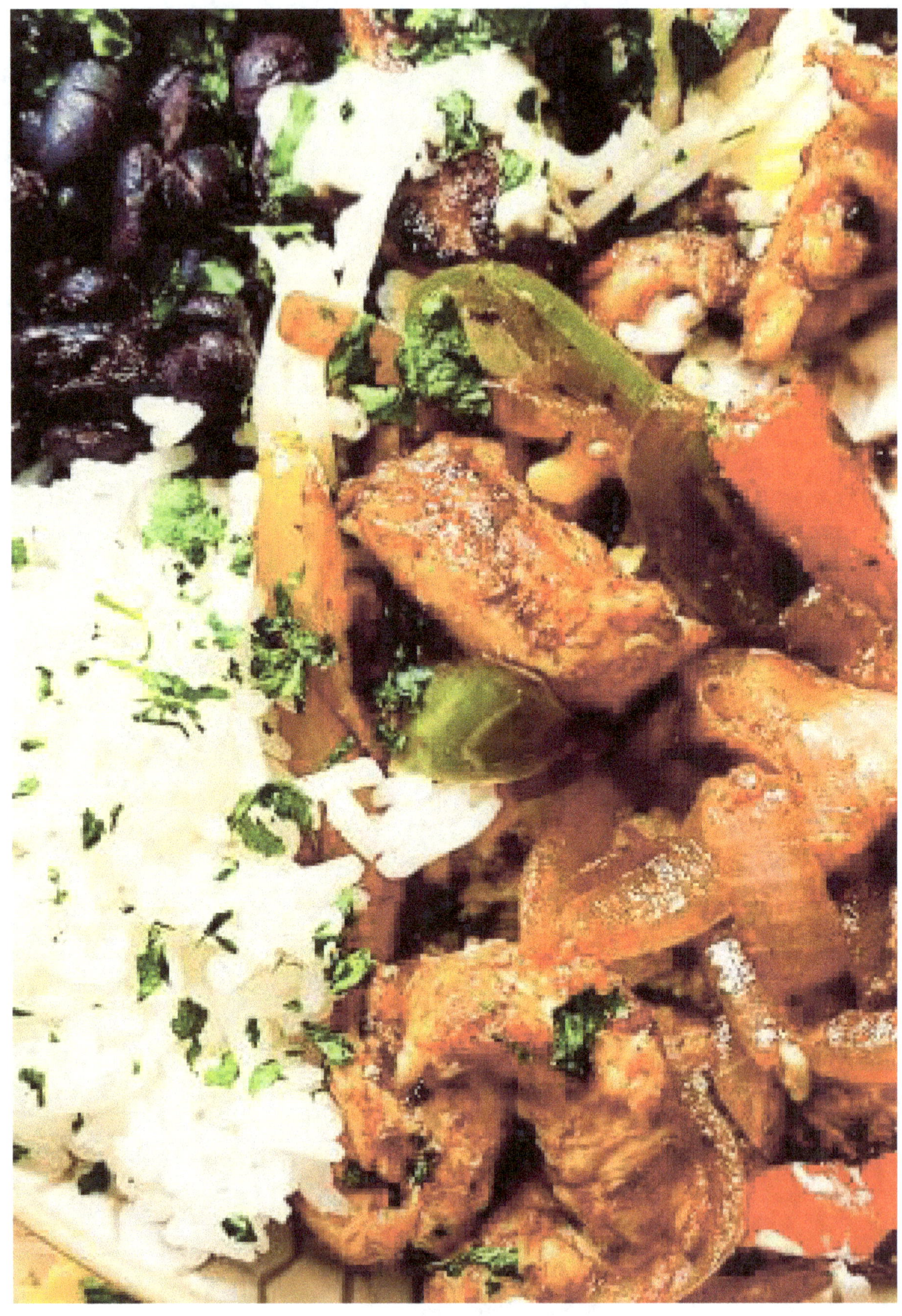

Joey Ramsey

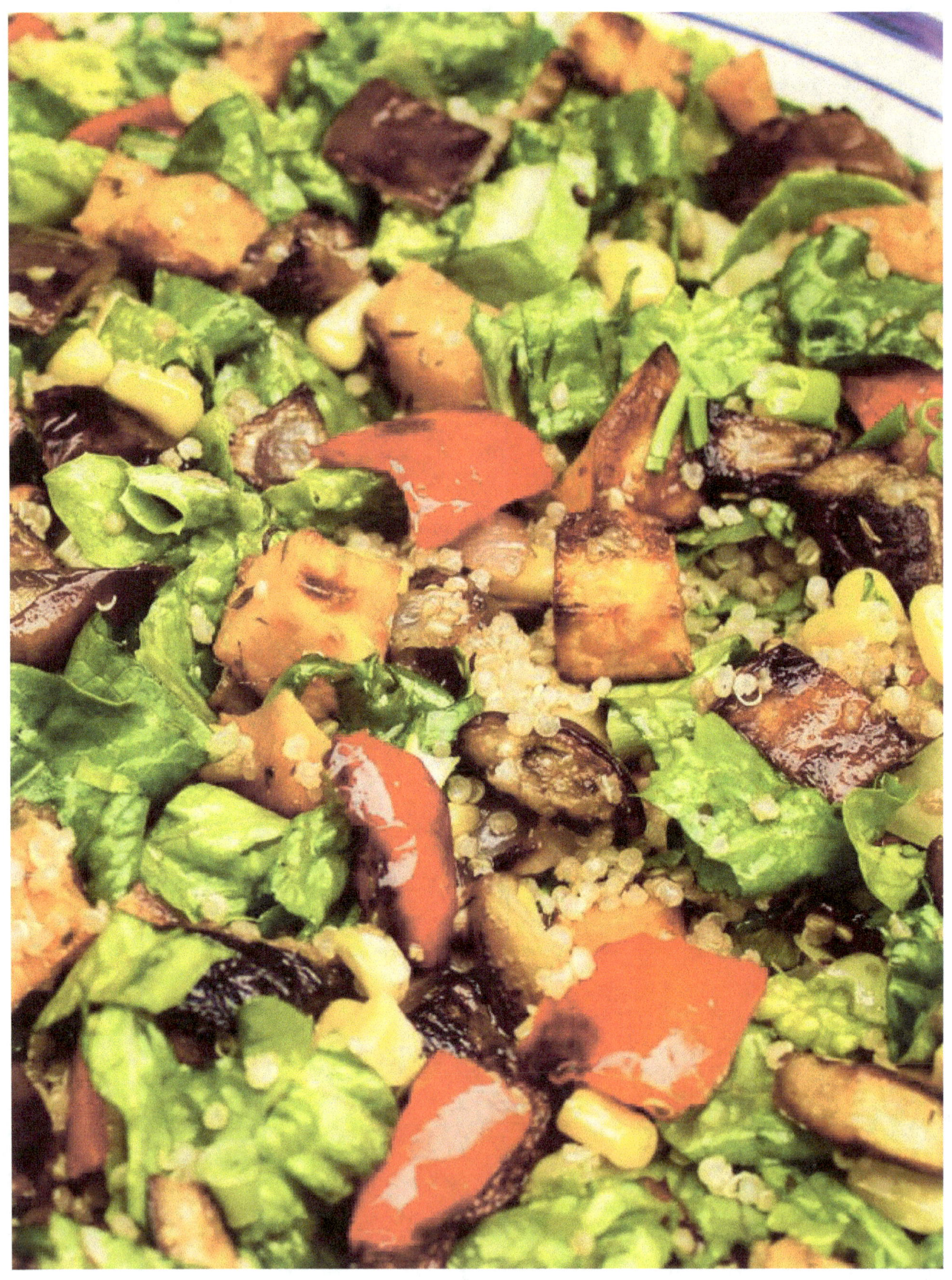

CONTENTS

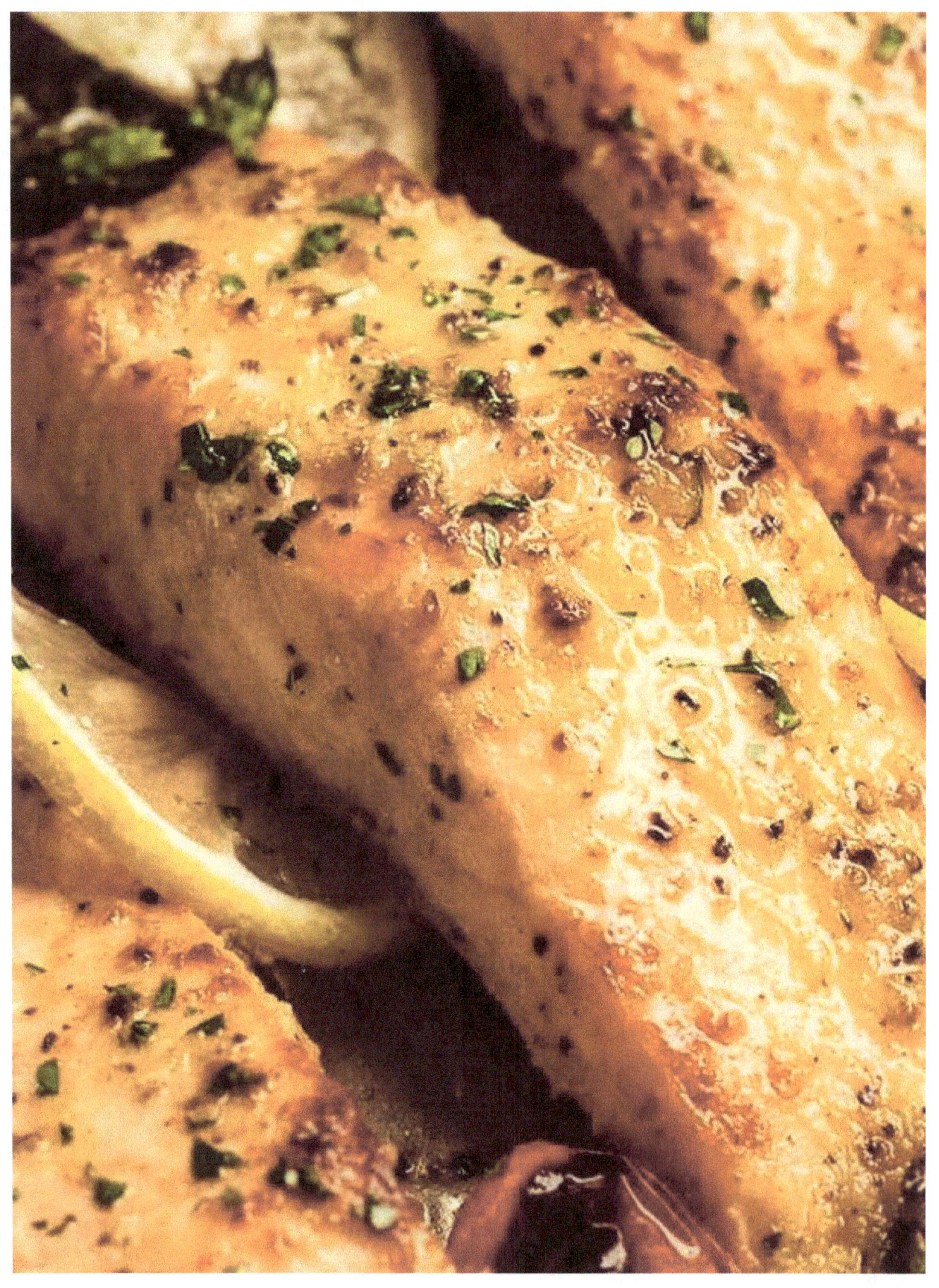

INTRODUCTION

About the Galveston Diet Cookbook

With my Detox Galveston Diet Cookbook there is the huge effect of hours of research, complete commitment and primary goal that is to promote the best health and wellness mainly during the life stage of menopause. Joey Ramsey has written the cookbook that applies the ground-breaking work of Dr. Mary Claire Haver, a well-known and respected expert on women's health and balanced hormones.

The start of writing this book by Joey Ramsey was the result of his close cousin's menopause and weight management problems. Just like many other women, she overcome the problems of hormonal changes and their effect on her built and her well-being. On the other hand, her devotion to Dr. Haver and his practices just lit up a fuse that broadened her view about health and nutrition.

By the means of thorough research and the application of Joey Ramsey principles, she not only succeeded in herself but also become enthusiastic about spreading this life-changing knowledge to others. Recognizing that the Galveston Diet had an extraordinary effect on her own health mission and determined to make the benefits of the diet available for women around the world, they decided to make it widely popular and accessible.

In Sarah's story we have an inspiration which is one evidence of the Galveston Diet transformative strength. Like many others, Sarah had weight management issues and also menopausal symptoms after a major life event- the loss of her mother to colon cancer. Although she tried to do some sports and control calories in her diet, she could not avoid weight gain related to menopause and other the signs of menopause.

Although it took Sarah the time and effort to discover the Galveston Diet and learn to apply its principles into her life style, the results were simply incredible. This was truly a remarkable change as it transformed her life within a period of 90 days. She lost seventeen (17) lb., reaching her goal weight and experiencing higher energy and reduction of hot flash. Her excitement about the program was felt, as she would gladly tell her friends about her success and search for opportunities to help other people to benefit from the science-based way of nutrition and wellness.

Sarah's story is a testimony that expresses the Galveston Diet's deep effect on women of today's generation and reminds us that we should opt for strategies backed by science in order to lead longer and healthier lives. His educational experience in nutrition represents another key aspect helping his novel to reach out to the widest number of people as it is a book which aims to educate people about the role of food in human health and encourages them to look after their health regardless of their level of knowledge about the subject.

The Galveston Diet Cookbook represents a vibrant convergence of the latest science with personal experience plus a deep commitment to empower women to prosper in their menopause and thereafter. Joey Ramsey's commitment and the stories of individuals such as Sarah that are inspiring, this cookbook is a symbol of hope and transformation for women who are looking for a way to healthy and energetic life.

How to Use This Cookbook

By acquiring the Galveston Diet Cookbook, you are giving yourself an opportunity to cook a range of delicious and nutritious recipes that are meant to be a power source for both your health and your wellness. Whether you are at the beginning of the Galveston Diet or you want to have more variety in your kitchen, this cookbook is your ultimate guide to nourishing meals that will both feed your body and your soul. Here's how to make the most of it:

❖ **Familiarize yourself with the Galveston Diet Principles:** Before going further into the recipes, let us first talk about the points of the Galveston Diet that serve as its foundation. As an evidence-based method, this protocol incorporates several important pillars, which involve hormone optimization, inflammation reduction, and a whole-food way of eating in order to address the many menopause related issues.

❖ **Explore the Recipe Categories:** The Galveston Diet Cookbook is divided into five categories: Breakfast, Lunch, Dinner, Snacks, and Desserts. Every part of the book has different recipes made according to your diet and your nutritional needs. If you are looking for a power packed breakfast, a full lunch or a reward dessert, you don't have to rummage through the options anymore.

❖ **Meal Planning:** Planning your meals is a crucial point in Galveston Diet development. Make some time each week to go through the cookbook, select the recipes that you like, and plan your meals for the week ahead. Look through for instance ingredient availability, prep time and dietary restrictions to make sure that meal prep is smooth and delicious.

❖ **Customize to Suit Your Taste:** Feel free to modify the recipes in order for them to perfectly match your taste and diet needs. No matter whether you are following a gluten-free, dairy-free, or vegetarian lifestyle, many of the recipes in this cookbook can be easily modified to fit your requirements. Try to vary herbs, spices, and combinations to make the dishes be uniquely yours.

❖ **Shop for Ingredients:** After you've decided on your meal plan, compose your list of ingredients and click it down at the grocery shop. Go for fresh, top quality ingredients anytime you can and don't hesitate to visit your local farmers' market for seasonal produce and artisanal products.

❖ **Prep and Cook with Care:** For the first step, we need to take time to collect all the required ingredients and equipment. Observation of the instructions is important, and you should not go too fast through the process of cooking. Cooking can be a therapeutic and enjoyable activity so just relax and enjoy the way.

❖ **Enjoy and Share Your Creations:** When your meal is done, just stand for a while and give your good looks and amazing smell to your creation. Sit down, take your time to taste every bite, and relish that satisfying feeling of having taken care of your physical and spiritual well-being. And don't forget to share your cooking masterpieces with your friends and family - they will be astonished by your newly acquired cooking skills!

❖ **Keep exploring and Learning:** The Galveston Diet Cookbook is only one step that will lay a foundation for your gourmet travel. Be willing to experiment with new recipes, ingredients, and cooking methods to make sure that your daily diet is exciting and your hunger is fulfilled. Keep on being curious, keep on being inspired and, above all, keep on being committed to feeding yourself and living the best life you can.

Galveston Diet Cookbook is not just a recipe collection, it is a practical tool to remaining well, happy, and healthy. If you keep in mind those tips and details you will be ready for well-balanced and scrumptious meals which help you to obtain your objectives and strengthen your body. To this happy cooking and a healthier, happier you!

Tips for Success

Starting a path toward a healthy life style, and the use of the Galveston Diet Cookbook as the tool for it, is both stimulating and inspiring.

❖ **Understand the Galveston Diet Principles:** First of all, prior to getting into the recipes, make sure that you are familiarized with the key components that make up the Galveston Diet. This science-driven technique highlights hormone optimization, inflammation reduction, and whole-food nutrition as the main tools for women's health, especially during menopause. The understanding of basic principles of the diet would better prepare you to correctly choose foods and hence, have your health goals.

❖ **Focus on Whole, Nutrient-Dense Foods:** The Galveston Diet's fundamental principle is eating whole, nutrient-dense foods which provides your body with abundant nourishment. Fresh fruits and vegetables, lean proteins, healthy fats, and whole grains should be your first choice in the meals. Besides, such quantities of essential vitamins and minerals can not only nourish your body but also help you stay full and filled with energy.

❖ **Prioritize Meal Planning and Preparation:** The other success factor for the Galveston diet is healthy meal preparation and planning. Don't forget to plan your meals for the week ahead, considering your schedule, your dietary preferences, and nutritional needs. The method of batch cooking and meal prepping can help you save the time you spend on cooking and thus your own homemade healthy meals would always be ready to enjoy whenever you get hungry.

❖ **Stay Hydrated:** The right amount of the water in the body is important for health and wellbeing, but then it is ignored. The aim is to drink a lot of water all day long to keep your body hydrated and to support the natural functions of your body. Herbal tea, infused water and coconut water can serve as some other great alternatives for hydration while making your beverage variety strong.

❖ **Listen to Your Body:** Mind your body's hunger and fullness sign, you eat mindfully without any diversions. Concentrate on relishing every mouthful, chewing slowly, and being aware of the way various foods affect you. Have a try at intuitive eating and tune your choices of food periodically so that what you get into your body is more what your body needs and prefers.

❖ **Incorporate Physical Activity:** Though nutrition is the primary factor in health, regular physical activity is also a part of a balanced approach to keep the body and mind fit. Locate little things that would excite you beyond walking, riding a bicycle, jogging or dancing and make movement a must in your daily schedule. Achieve an optimal fitness result by integrating various types of workouts which include cardio exercise, weight or muscle building exercise and flexibility activity.

❖ **Practice Self-Care and Stress Management:** The management of stress and the provision of self-care are the key elements of a balanced life. Include relaxation therapy techniques for example, meditation, deep breathing exercises and mindfulness practices in your daily routine to reduce stress which ultimately leads to overall health. Recall to have ample sleep at the end of the day, to relax and to have pleasurable activities since they also energize and recharge your body and mind.

❖ **Stay Consistent and Patient:** The process of maintaining the gained results is long, and it requires a lot of time, consistency, and patience. Be rational while assessing your level of expectation, and congratulate yourself even on the tiniest success marks. Remember that you are making a positive choice for each step you are taking, regardless of the size, for your own good and well-being so always stay focused on your goal and trust in the process.

With these tips you will be ready to start your Galveston Diet journey with confidence and enthusiasm. Be mindful that each measure of your journey towards heightened health and overall wellness is priceless, and you deserve to live a fulfilling life. While feeling better isn't a guarantee, it's worth a try to achieve a more joyful and well-being state of mind!

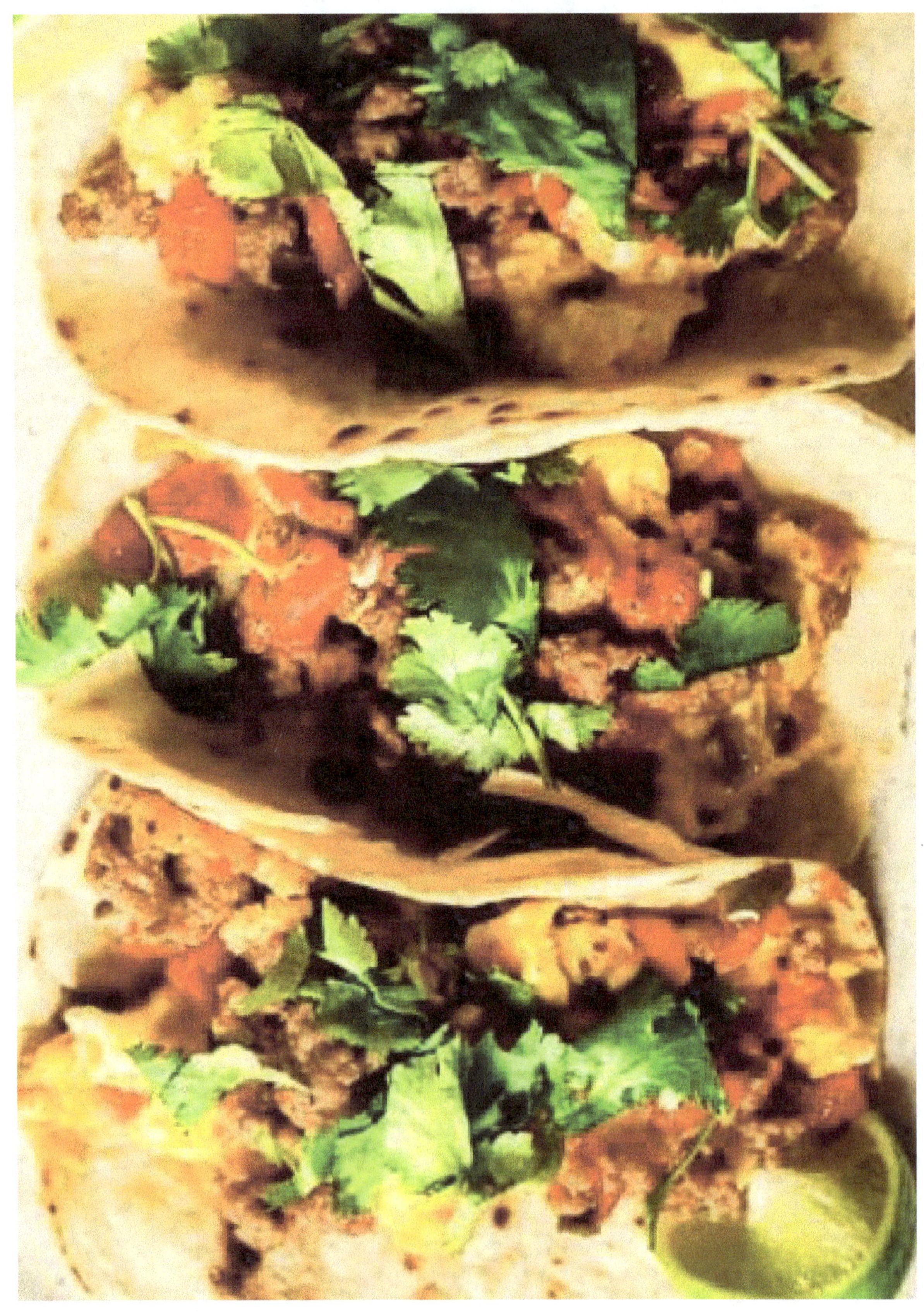

Joey Ramsey

1

BREAKFAST RECIPES

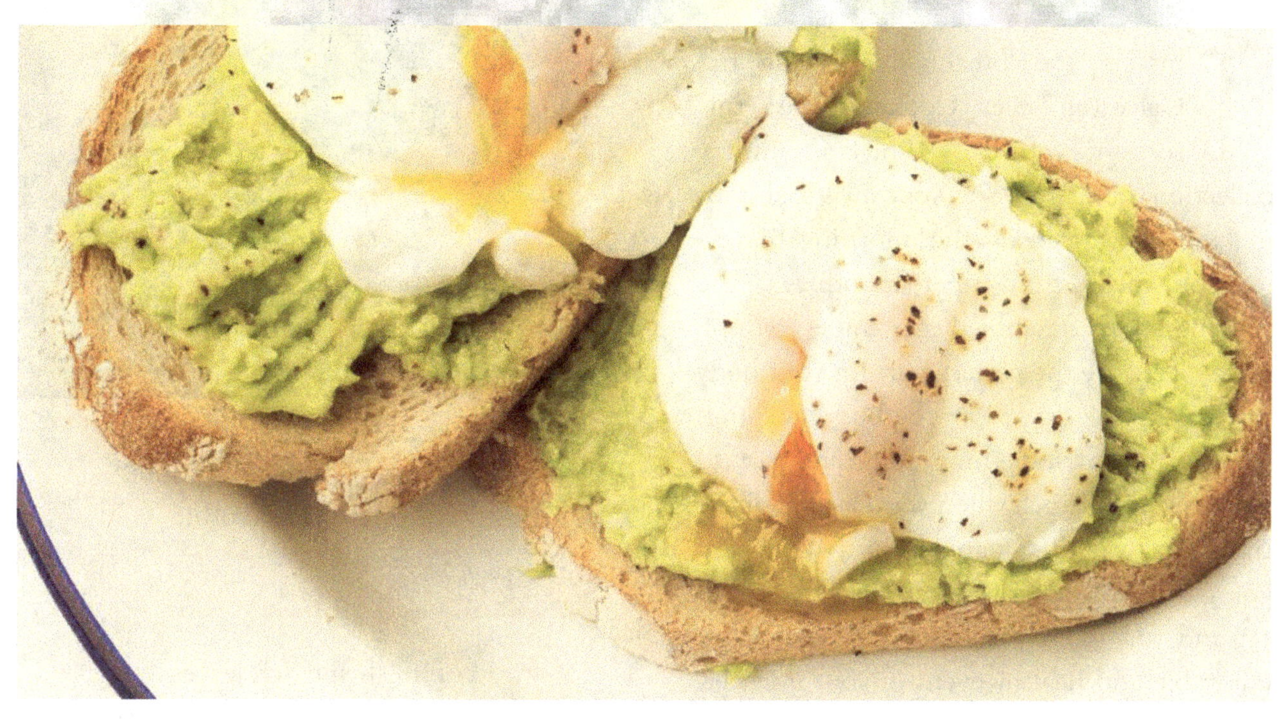

A Delicious Start to Your Day

Galveston Green Smoothie

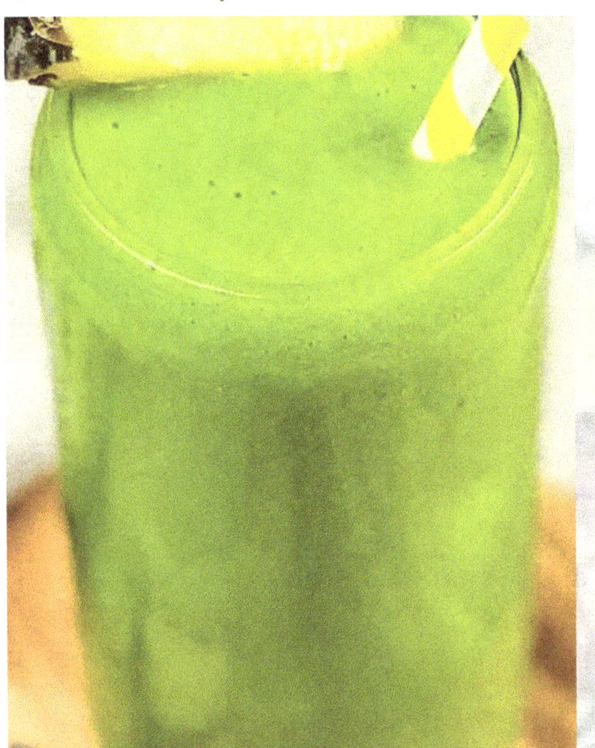

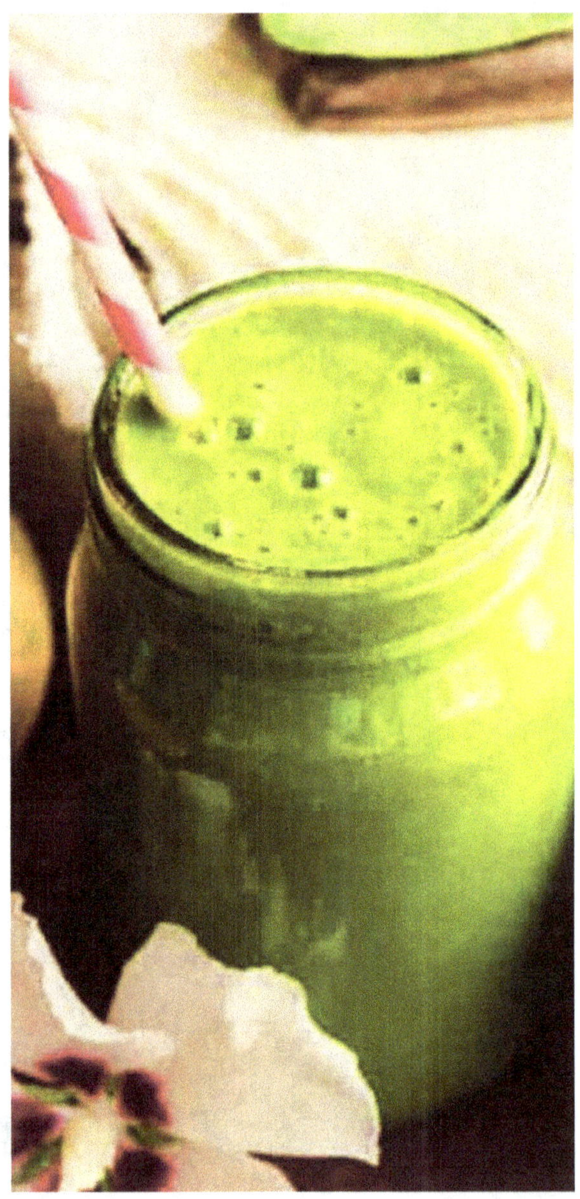

This is the breakfast part of the Galveston Diet Cookbook. In this section you will find a yummy collection of recipes for your new habit of making the most of the morning. These delicious meals, from super smoothies to the protein-packed scrambled eggs and everything in between, are the perfect start for your body to conquer the day. From the busy mornings when you want something quick and easy to the weekend brunch when you have plenty of time, you will find many ideas to keep you going through the day. Hence, get the apron on and turn your breakfast routine into an enjoyable and healthy event in your everyday life.

- ❖ **Preparation Time:** 5 minutes
- ❖ **Serving Unit:** 1 smoothie

Ingredients:

- ❖ 1 cup fresh spinach leaves
- ❖ ½ ripe avocado, peeled and pitted
- ❖ ½ cup frozen pineapple chunks
- ❖ ½ cup frozen mango chunks

- ❖ 1 tablespoon chia seeds
- ❖ 1 tablespoon honey or maple syrup (optional)
- ❖ 1 cup unsweetened almond milk or coconut water
- ❖ Ice cubes (optional)

Procedures:

- ❖ In a blender, combine the fresh spinach leaves, ripe avocado, frozen pineapple chunks, frozen mango chunks, chia seeds, and honey or maple syrup (if using).
- ❖ Pour in the unsweetened almond milk or coconut water.
- ❖ Blend on high speed until smooth and creamy, adding ice cubes if desired for a colder consistency.
- ❖ Once thoroughly blended, pour the smoothie into a glass and serve immediately.

Nutritional Value (per serving):

- ❖ **Calories:** 290 kcal
- ❖ **Protein:** 6g
- ❖ **Fat:** 14g
- ❖ **Carbohydrates:** 38g
- ❖ **Fiber:** 12g
- ❖ **Sugar:** 20g
- ❖ **Vitamin A:** 90% DV
- ❖ **Vitamin C:** 120% DV
- ❖ **Calcium:** 35% DV
- ❖ **Iron:** 25% DV

Cooking Tips:

- ❖ For a thicker consistency, use frozen spinach instead of fresh, or add additional avocado.
- ❖ Customize the sweetness of the smoothie by adjusting the amount of honey or maple syrup to suit your taste preferences.
- ❖ Experiment with different greens such as kale or Swiss chard for variety and added nutrients.
- ❖ To make the smoothie more filling, add a scoop of protein powder or Greek yogurt.

Health Benefits:

- ❖ **Rich in Nutrients:** This green smoothie is packed with vitamins, minerals, and antioxidants from the spinach, avocado, pineapple, and mango, providing essential nutrients for overall health and well-being.
- ❖ **Good Source of Fiber:** With the addition of chia seeds and fiber-rich fruits, this smoothie is an excellent source of dietary fiber, promoting digestive health and helping you feel full and satisfied.
- ❖ **Heart-Healthy Fats:** The avocado contributes heart-healthy monounsaturated fats, which may help lower cholesterol levels and reduce the risk of heart disease.
- ❖ **Hydrating:** Coconut water or almond milk adds hydration to the smoothie, keeping you refreshed and replenished.
- ❖ **Supports Immune Function:** The high vitamin C content from the fruits

boosts immune function and helps protect against infections and illnesses.

* **Energy Boost:** This smoothie provides a natural energy boost to start your day, thanks to the combination of carbohydrates, healthy fats, and vitamins.

The Galveston Green Smoothie is not only beneficial, it is also a tasty way for you to start your day and give your body neatly packed nutrients. With the rejuvenating green color and luscious taste of this smoothie, it is bound to be a breakfast staple that provides you with that fresh feeling throughout the morning.

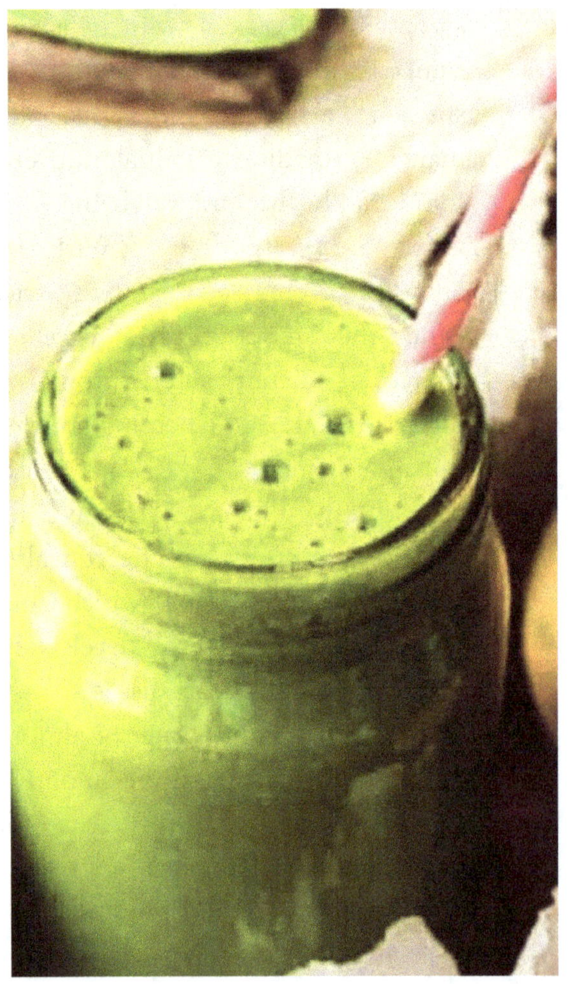

Tex-Mex Breakfast Casserole

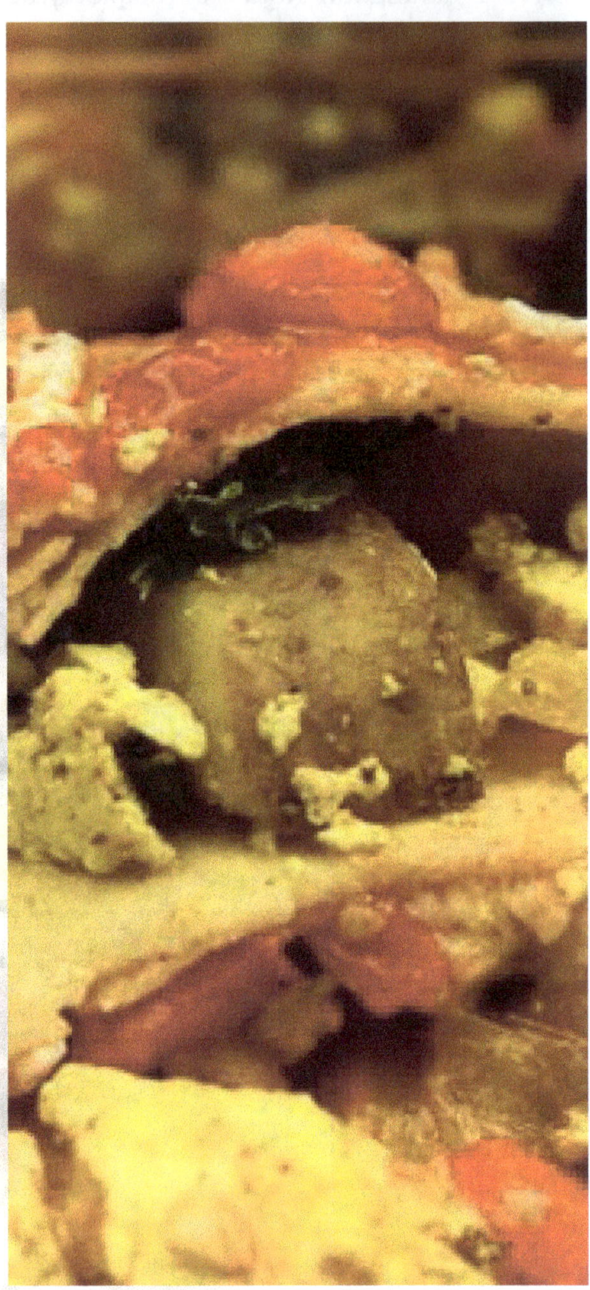

* **Preparation Time:** 15 minutes
* **Cooking Time:** 45 minutes
* **Serving Unit:** 6 servings

Ingredients:

* 8 large eggs
* ½ cup milk (dairy or non-dairy)

- ❖ 1 teaspoon chili powder
- ❖ ½ teaspoon cumin
- ❖ ½ teaspoon garlic powder
- ❖ Salt and pepper, to taste
- ❖ 6 corn tortillas, torn into bite-sized pieces
- ❖ 1 cup cooked black beans
- ❖ 1 cup diced bell peppers (any color)
- ❖ 1 cup diced tomatoes
- ❖ 1 cup shredded cheddar cheese
- ❖ ¼ cup chopped fresh cilantro (optional)
- ❖ Salsa, avocado, and Greek yogurt, for serving (optional)

Procedures:

- ❖ Preheat the oven to 375°F (190°C). Grease a 9x13-inch baking dish with cooking spray or oil.
- ❖ In a large mixing bowl, whisk together the eggs, milk, chili powder, cumin, garlic powder, salt, and pepper until well combined.
- ❖ Spread half of the torn corn tortillas evenly across the bottom of the prepared baking dish.
- ❖ Layer half of the black beans, bell peppers, tomatoes, and shredded cheese over the tortillas.
- ❖ Pour half of the egg mixture over the layered ingredients in the baking dish.
- ❖ Repeat the layering process with the remaining tortillas, black beans, bell peppers, tomatoes, cheese, and egg mixture.
- ❖ Cover the baking dish with foil and bake in the preheated oven for 30 minutes.

- ❖ Remove the foil and continue baking for an additional 15 minutes, or until the casserole is set and the top is lightly golden brown.
- ❖ Once cooked through, remove the casserole from the oven and let it cool for a few minutes before slicing.
- ❖ Garnish with chopped cilantro, if desired, and serve warm with salsa, avocado, and Greek yogurt on the side.

Nutritional Value (per serving):

- ❖ **Calories:** 320 kcal
- ❖ **Protein:** 20g
- ❖ **Fat:** 15g
- ❖ **Carbohydrates:** 25g
- ❖ **Fiber:** 5g
- ❖ **Sugar:** 3g

Cooking Tips:

- ❖ Customize the casserole by adding cooked breakfast sausage, diced ham, or crumbled bacon for extra protein and flavor.
- ❖ Make it spicy by adding diced jalapeños or a dash of hot sauce to the egg mixture.
- ❖ For a vegetarian option, omit the meat and add more vegetables such as mushrooms, spinach, or onions.
- ❖ Make ahead: Prepare the casserole the night before, cover, and refrigerate overnight. In the morning, simply bake as directed, adding a few extra minutes to the cooking time if needed.

Health Benefits:

- ❖ **High Protein:** Eggs are a rich source of high-quality protein, which is essential for building and repairing tissues, as well as supporting muscle health.
- ❖ **Fiber-Rich:** Black beans and vegetables provide dietary fiber, which aids in digestion, promotes satiety, and helps regulate blood sugar levels.
- ❖ **Vitamins and Minerals:** Bell peppers and tomatoes are packed with vitamins A and C, as well as potassium and other essential nutrients, which support immune function and overall health.
- ❖ **Healthy Fats:** Avocado, cheese, and eggs contribute healthy fats that are important for brain function, hormone production, and heart health.
- ❖ **Balanced Meal:** This Tex-Mex breakfast casserole offers a balance of protein, carbohydrates, and fats, making it a satisfying and nourishing option to start your day.

Tex-Mex Breakfast Casserole is a flavorful and nutritious dish that is perfect for feeding a crowd or meal prepping for busy mornings. With its combination of protein-rich eggs, fiber-packed beans and vegetables, and zesty Tex-Mex flavors, it's sure to become a breakfast favorite that everyone will love. Enjoy it as is or customize it to suit your taste preferences— it's versatile, delicious, and packed with health benefits.

Coconut Flour Pancakes with Berries

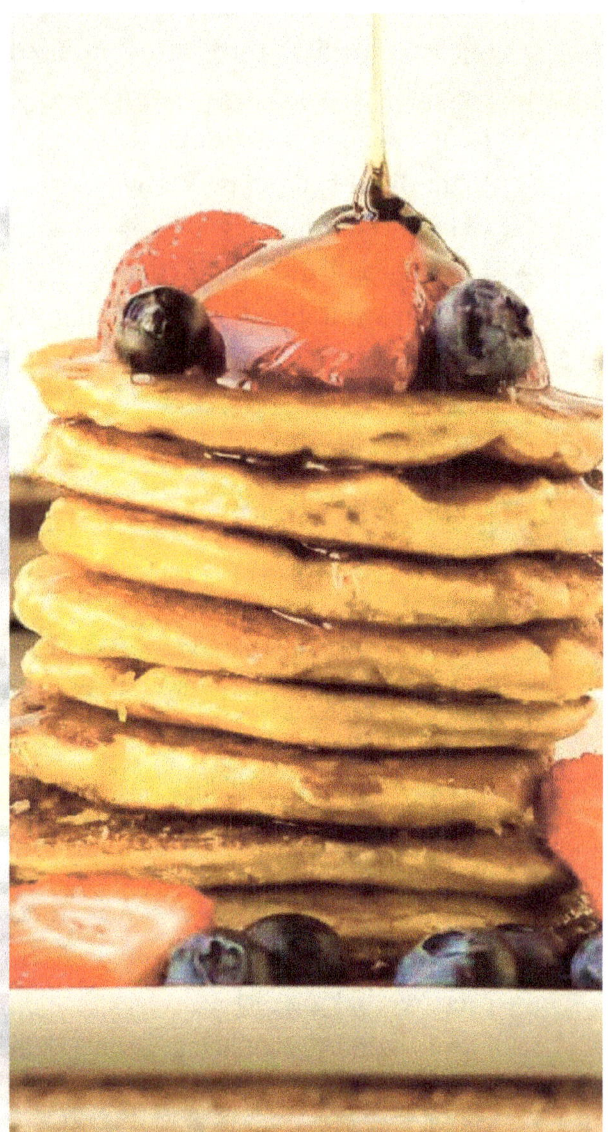

- ❖ **Preparation Time:** 10 minutes
- ❖ **Cooking Time:** 15 minutes
- ❖ **Serving Unit:** Makes 8 pancakes

Ingredients:

- ❖ 4 large eggs
- ❖ ½ cup coconut milk
- ❖ ¼ cup coconut oil, melted

❖ 1 teaspoon vanilla extract
❖ ¼ cup coconut flour
❖ 1 teaspoon baking powder
❖ Pinch of salt
❖ Fresh berries (such as strawberries, blueberries, raspberries) for serving
❖ Maple syrup or honey for serving

Procedures:

❖ In a large mixing bowl, whisk together the eggs, coconut milk, melted coconut oil, and vanilla extract until well combined.
❖ In a separate bowl, sift together the coconut flour, baking powder, and salt.
❖ Gradually add the dry ingredients to the wet ingredients, whisking until a smooth batter forms. Let the batter rest for a few minutes to allow the coconut flour to absorb the liquid.
❖ Heat a non-stick skillet or griddle over medium heat and lightly grease with coconut oil or cooking spray.
❖ Spoon about ¼ cup of batter onto the skillet for each pancake, spreading it out slightly with the back of the spoon.
❖ Cook for 2-3 minutes, or until bubbles start to form on the surface of the pancake and the edges begin to set.
❖ Carefully flip the pancake and cook for an additional 1-2 minutes on the other side, until golden brown and cooked through.
❖ Repeat with the remaining batter, adjusting the heat as needed to prevent burning.
❖ Serve the pancakes warm, topped with fresh berries and drizzled with maple syrup or honey.

Nutritional Value (per serving, without toppings):

❖ **Calories:** 140 kcal
❖ **Protein:** 4g
❖ **Fat:** 11g
❖ **Carbohydrates:** 6g
❖ **Fiber:** 3g
❖ **Sugar:** 1g

Cooking Tips:

❖ Coconut flour tends to absorb a lot of liquid, so the batter may thicken as it sits. If necessary, add a little extra coconut milk to achieve the desired consistency.
❖ For lighter and fluffier pancakes, separate the egg yolks from the whites. Whisk the yolks into the batter as directed, then beat the egg whites until stiff peaks form. Gently fold the beaten egg whites into the batter just before cooking.
❖ To prevent sticking, ensure that your skillet or griddle is well-greased before adding the batter. Use a non-stick surface or a well-seasoned cast iron skillet for best results.
❖ Keep the pancakes warm while cooking the remaining batches by placing them on a baking sheet in a preheated oven set to low heat.

Health Benefits:

- ❖ **Gluten-Free:** Coconut flour is naturally gluten-free, making these pancakes suitable for individuals with gluten sensitivities or celiac disease.
- ❖ **High in Fiber:** Coconut flour is rich in dietary fiber, which promotes digestive health, helps regulate blood sugar levels, and contributes to feelings of fullness and satiety.
- ❖ **Healthy Fats:** Coconut milk and coconut oil provide healthy fats, including medium-chain triglycerides (MCTs), which are easily digested and may support weight management and brain health.
- ❖ **Protein-Rich:** Eggs are a good source of high-quality protein, which is essential for muscle repair and growth, as well as overall health and vitality.
- ❖ **Antioxidant-Rich:** Fresh berries are loaded with antioxidants, vitamins, and minerals, which help protect against oxidative stress, inflammation, and chronic disease.

Coconut Flour Pancakes with Berries are a delicious and nutritious option for a wholesome breakfast or brunch. With their light and fluffy texture, subtle coconut flavor, and vibrant berry toppings, they're sure to delight your taste buds and nourish your body. Enjoy them as a guilt-free indulgence any day of the week!

Southwest Breakfast Tacos

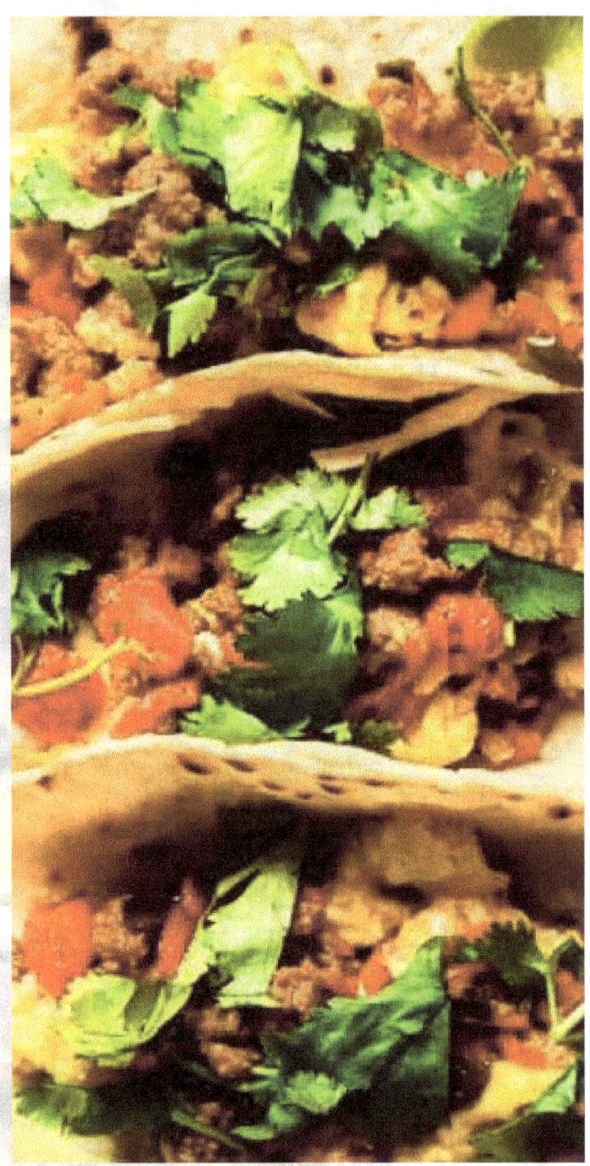

- ❖ **Preparation Time:** 15 minutes
- ❖ **Cooking Time:** 10 minutes
- ❖ **Serving Unit:** Makes 4 tacos

Ingredients:

- ❖ 4 large eggs
- ❖ 1 tablespoon olive oil
- ❖ ½ cup diced bell peppers (any color)
- ❖ ½ cup diced onion

* ½ cup black beans, drained and rinsed
* ½ teaspoon chili powder
* ½ teaspoon cumin
* Salt and pepper, to taste
* 4 small whole wheat or corn tortillas
* ½ cup shredded cheddar cheese
* Fresh cilantro, diced avocado, salsa, and Greek yogurt for serving (optional)

Procedures:

* In a small bowl, whisk together the eggs until well beaten. Set aside.
* In a large skillet, heat the olive oil over medium heat. Add the diced bell peppers and onions, and sauté until softened, about 3-4 minutes.
* Add the black beans to the skillet, along with the chili powder, cumin, salt, and pepper. Cook for an additional 2-3 minutes, stirring occasionally.
* Push the vegetables and beans to one side of the skillet and pour the beaten eggs into the empty space. Cook, stirring gently, until the eggs are scrambled and cooked through, about 2-3 minutes.
* Warm the tortillas in a separate skillet or in the microwave until soft and pliable.
* To assemble the tacos, spoon the egg mixture onto each tortilla, then sprinkle with shredded cheddar cheese. Top with fresh cilantro, diced avocado, salsa, and Greek yogurt, if desired.
* Fold the tortillas in half or roll them up tightly, and serve immediately.

Nutritional Value (per serving, without optional toppings):

* **Calories:** 240 kcal
* **Protein:** 12g
* **Fat:** 10g
* **Carbohydrates:** 25g
* **Fiber:** 6g
* **Sugar:** 3g

Cooking Tips:

* Customize the filling by adding cooked breakfast sausage, diced ham, or crumbled bacon for extra flavor and protein.
* Feel free to use any variety of bell peppers or onions that you have on hand, or substitute with other vegetables such as mushrooms, spinach, or tomatoes.
* For a spicier kick, add a dash of hot sauce or a sprinkle of crushed red pepper flakes to the egg mixture.
* If using corn tortillas, heat them briefly over an open flame or in a dry skillet before assembling the tacos to enhance their flavor and texture.

Health Benefits:

* **High Protein:** Eggs are a rich source of high-quality protein, which is essential for muscle repair and growth, as well as overall health and vitality.
* **Fiber-Rich:** Black beans and vegetables provide dietary fiber, which

promotes digestive health, helps regulate blood sugar levels, and contributes to feelings of fullness and satiety.

❖ **Healthy Fats:** Olive oil and avocado contribute heart-healthy monounsaturated fats, which may help lower cholesterol levels and reduce the risk of heart disease.

❖ **Nutrient-Dense:** Bell peppers and onions are packed with vitamins, minerals, and antioxidants, including vitamin C and vitamin A, which support immune function and overall health.

❖ **Low-Glycemic:** Whole wheat or corn tortillas provide complex carbohydrates that are digested more slowly, helping to maintain steady blood sugar levels and prevent energy crashes.

These **Southwest Breakfast Tacos** are a delicious and satisfying way to start your day on a nutritious note. With their flavorful egg and veggie filling, cheesy goodness, and customizable toppings, they're sure to become a breakfast favorite that you'll want to enjoy again and again. Serve them up for a leisurely weekend brunch or whip them up for a quick and easy weekday meal—either way, they're bound to impress!

Avocado Toast with Poached Egg

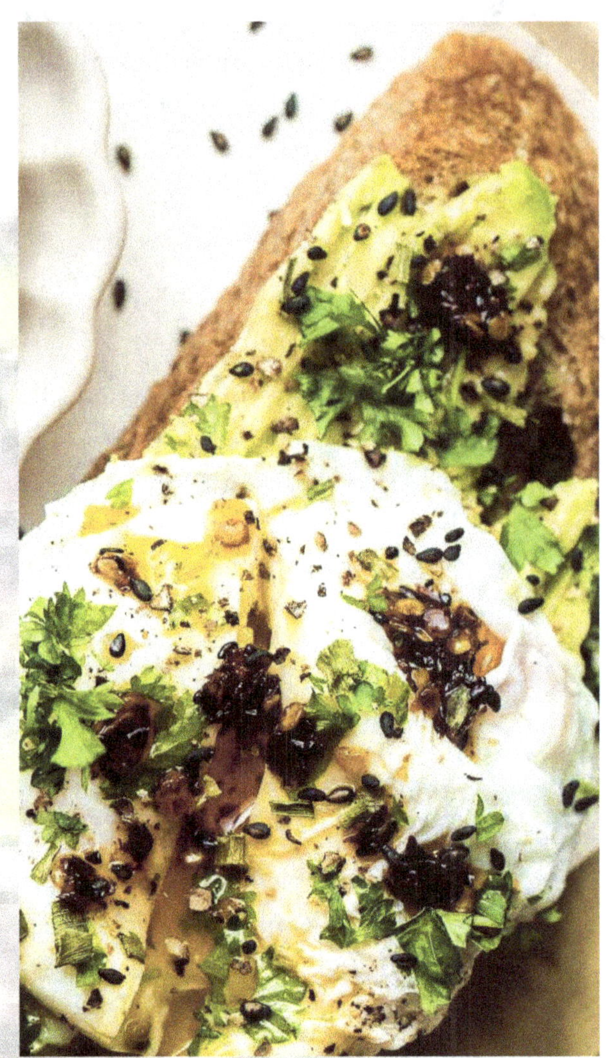

❖ **Preparation Time:** 10 minutes
❖ **Cooking Time:** 5 minutes
❖ **Serving Unit:** Makes 2 servings

Ingredients:

❖ 2 large eggs
❖ 2 slices whole grain bread, toasted
❖ 1 ripe avocado
❖ 1 teaspoon lemon juice
❖ Salt and pepper, to taste

- ❖ Red pepper flakes, for garnish (optional)
- ❖ Fresh herbs (such as cilantro or parsley), for garnish (optional)
- ❖ Cherry tomatoes, sliced, for serving (optional)

Procedures:

- ❖ Fill a medium-sized saucepan with water and bring it to a gentle simmer over medium heat.
- ❖ Crack one egg into a small bowl or ramekin, taking care not to break the yolk. Use a spoon to create a gentle whirlpool in the simmering water.
- ❖ Carefully slide the egg into the center of the whirlpool and let it cook for 3-4 minutes, until the whites are set but the yolk is still runny. Use a slotted spoon to carefully remove the poached egg from the water and transfer it to a plate lined with paper towels to drain. Repeat the process with the second egg.
- ❖ While the eggs are poaching, prepare the avocado. Cut the avocado in half lengthwise and remove the pit. Scoop the flesh into a small bowl and mash it with a fork until smooth. Stir in the lemon juice, salt, and pepper to taste.
- ❖ Spread the mashed avocado evenly onto the toasted slices of bread.
- ❖ Carefully place a poached egg on top of each piece of avocado toast.
- ❖ Garnish with red pepper flakes, fresh herbs, and sliced cherry tomatoes, if desired.

- ❖ Serve immediately, while the egg yolk is still warm and runny.

Nutritional Value (per serving):

- ❖ **Calories:** 270 kcal
- ❖ **Protein:** 11g
- ❖ **Fat:** 17g
- ❖ **Carbohydrates:** 21g
- ❖ **Fiber:** 8g
- ❖ **Sugar:** 2g

Cooking Tips:

- ❖ Use fresh, ripe avocados for the best flavor and texture. You'll know an avocado is ripe when it yields slightly too gentle pressure when squeezed.
- ❖ To prevent the avocado from browning, add lemon juice or lime juice to the mashed avocado. This not only adds flavor but also helps preserve the vibrant green color.
- ❖ For perfectly poached eggs, use fresh eggs and ensure the water is at a gentle simmer—not boiling—before adding the eggs. Adding a splash of vinegar to the water can help the egg whites coagulate faster.
- ❖ To customize your avocado toast, try adding additional toppings such as sliced radishes, arugula, feta cheese, or smoked salmon.

Health Benefits:

- ❖ **Heart-Healthy Fats:** Avocado is a rich source of monounsaturated fats, which have been linked to improved heart health and reduced inflammation.

- ❖ **Protein-Rich:** Eggs are packed with high-quality protein, essential for muscle repair and growth, as well as overall health and vitality.
- ❖ **Fiber-Dense:** Whole grain bread provides dietary fiber, which aids in digestion, promotes satiety, and helps regulate blood sugar levels.
- ❖ **Nutrient-Packed:** Avocado is loaded with vitamins, minerals, and antioxidants, including vitamins E, K, and B-vitamins, as well as potassium and folate.
- ❖ **Low-Glycemic:** Whole grain bread has a lower glycemic index compared to refined grains, meaning it causes a slower and steadier rise in blood sugar levels.

Avocado Toast with Poached Egg is a simple yet satisfying breakfast option that's bursting with flavor and nutrition. With its creamy avocado, perfectly poached egg, and crunchy whole grain bread, it's a delicious way to start your day on a wholesome note. Whip it up for a leisurely weekend brunch or enjoy it as a quick and nutritious weekday meal—the choice is yours!

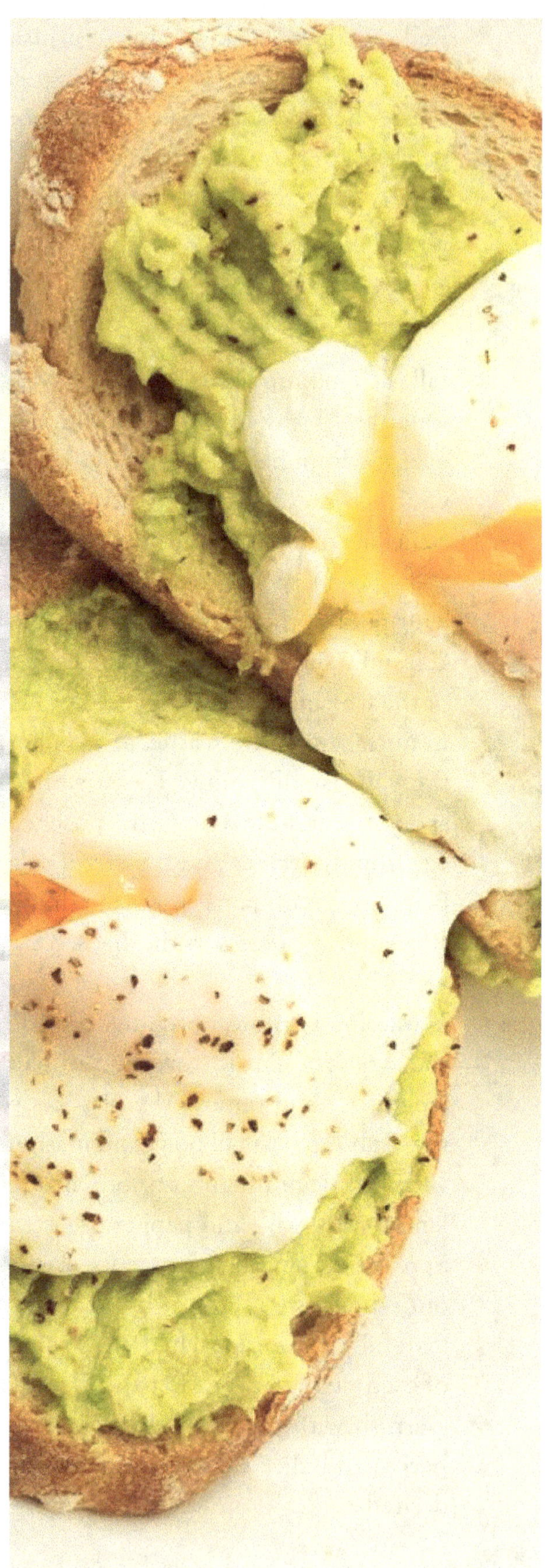

2

LUNCH RECIPES

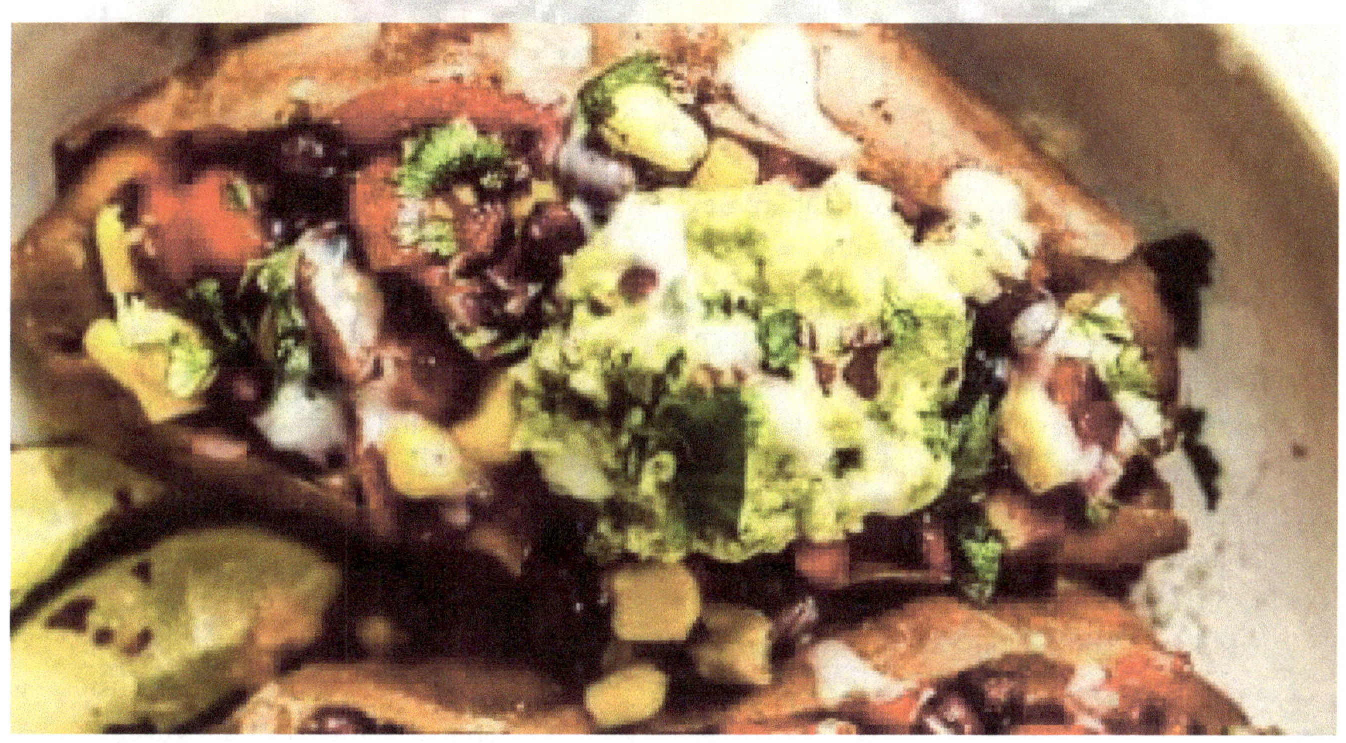

Delicious Midday Meals

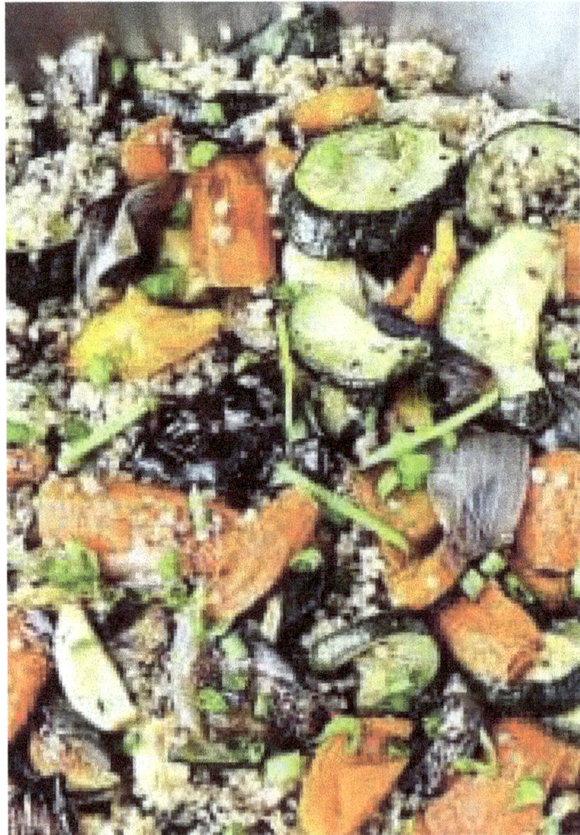

Grilled Shrimp Salad with Citrus Dressing

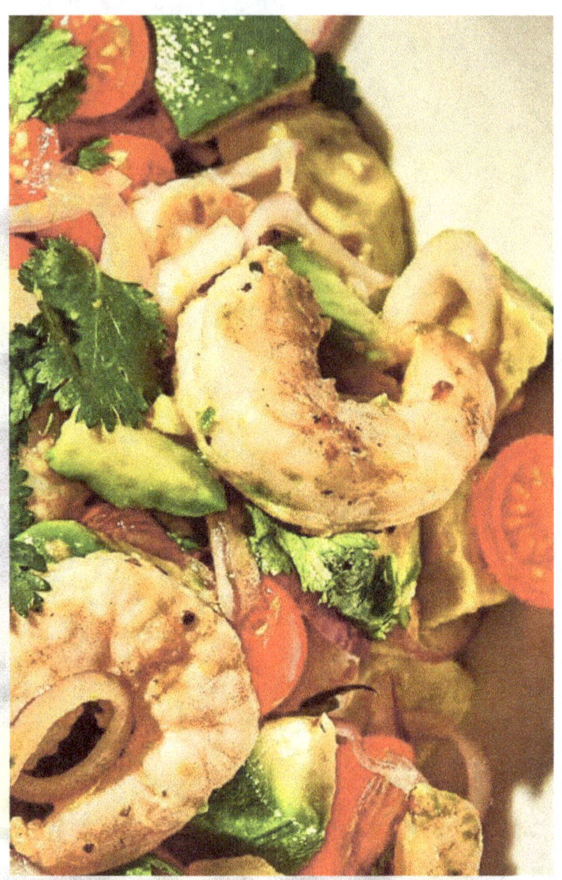

Welcome to the lunch section of the Galveston Diet Cookbook! Here, you'll discover a variety of mouthwatering recipes to fuel your afternoon and keep you satisfied until dinner. From hearty salads and nourishing soups to satisfying wraps and sandwiches, these lunch recipes are designed to provide a balance of nutrients and flavors to support your health and wellness goals. Whether you're meal-prepping for the week ahead or enjoying a leisurely lunch at home, you'll find plenty of inspiration to elevate your midday meal. So, let's dive in and explore the delicious options awaiting you in this section!

❖ **Preparation Time:** 20 minutes
❖ **Cooking Time:** 5 minutes
❖ **Serving Unit:** Makes 4 servings

Ingredients:

❖ 1 pound large shrimp, peeled and deveined
❖ 2 tablespoons olive oil
❖ 1 teaspoon smoked paprika
❖ ½ teaspoon garlic powder
❖ Salt and pepper, to taste
❖ 6 cups mixed salad greens (such as spinach, arugula, and lettuce)
❖ 1 cup cherry tomatoes, halved

- ❖ ½ cup sliced cucumber
- ❖ ¼ cup sliced red onion
- ❖ 1 avocado, diced
- ❖ ¼ cup chopped fresh cilantro or parsley

For the Citrus Dressing:

- ❖ ¼ cup freshly squeezed orange juice
- ❖ 2 tablespoons freshly squeezed lemon juice
- ❖ 1 tablespoon honey or maple syrup
- ❖ 1 teaspoon Dijon mustard
- ❖ ¼ cup olive oil
- ❖ Salt and pepper, to taste

Procedures:

- ❖ Preheat a grill or grill pan over medium-high heat. In a mixing bowl, toss the shrimp with olive oil, smoked paprika, garlic powder, salt, and pepper until evenly coated.
- ❖ Thread the seasoned shrimp onto skewers, if using, to make them easier to grill.
- ❖ Grill the shrimp for 2-3 minutes per side, or until they are pink and opaque. Remove from the grill and set aside.
- ❖ In a large salad bowl, combine the mixed greens, cherry tomatoes, sliced cucumber, red onion, avocado, and chopped cilantro or parsley.
- ❖ In a small jar or bowl, whisk together the orange juice, lemon juice, honey or maple syrup, Dijon mustard, olive oil, salt, and pepper to make the citrus dressing.

- ❖ Drizzle the citrus dressing over the salad and toss gently to coat the ingredients evenly.
- ❖ Divide the salad among serving plates and top each with grilled shrimp skewers.
- ❖ Serve immediately, garnished with additional fresh herbs if desired.

Nutritional Value (per serving):

- ❖ **Calories:** 310 kcal
- ❖ **Protein:** 20g
- ❖ **Fat:** 20g
- ❖ **Carbohydrates:** 18g
- ❖ **Fiber:** 6g
- ❖ **Sugar:** 8g

Cooking Tips:

- ❖ To prevent shrimp from sticking to the grill, make sure it is well-oiled and preheated before adding the shrimp. You can also use a grill pan or grill basket lined with aluminum foil for easier cleanup.
- ❖ Don't overcook the shrimp, as they can become tough and rubbery. Grill them just until they turn pink and opaque, about 2-3 minutes per side depending on their size.
- ❖ Customize the salad with your favorite vegetables and greens. Feel free to add or substitute ingredients such as bell peppers, carrots, radishes, or baby kale.
- ❖ For added flavor and texture, consider adding crumbled feta cheese, toasted nuts or seeds, or sliced avocado to the salad.

Health Benefits:

- ❖ **Lean Protein:** Shrimp is a low-calorie, high-protein food that provides essential nutrients such as selenium, vitamin B12, and omega-3 fatty acids, which support heart health and muscle repair.
- ❖ **Nutrient-Rich Greens:** Mixed salad greens are packed with vitamins, minerals, and antioxidants, including vitamins A, C, and K, folate, and potassium, which promote overall health and well-being.
- ❖ **Healthy Fats:** Olive oil and avocado contribute heart-healthy monounsaturated fats, which may help lower cholesterol levels and reduce the risk of heart disease.
- ❖ **Antioxidant-Packed:** Citrus fruits such as oranges and lemons are rich in vitamin C and other antioxidants, which help protect against oxidative stress and inflammation.
- ❖ **Fiber-Filled:** Vegetables like cherry tomatoes, cucumber, and red onion provide dietary fiber, which aids in digestion, promotes satiety, and helps regulate blood sugar levels.

This **Grilled Shrimp Salad with Citrus Dressing** is a light yet satisfying meal that's bursting with flavor and nutrition. With its succulent grilled shrimp, crisp mixed greens, and vibrant citrus dressing, it's the perfect dish for a refreshing summer lunch or dinner. Whip it up for a quick and healthy meal that's sure to impress!

Quinoa Salad with Roasted Vegetables

- ❖ **Preparation Time:** 15 minutes
- ❖ **Cooking Time:** 25 minutes
- ❖ **Serving Unit:** Makes 4 servings

Ingredients:

- ❖ 1 cup quinoa, rinsed
- ❖ 2 cups water or vegetable broth
- ❖ 1 tablespoon olive oil
- ❖ 2 cups mixed vegetables (such as bell peppers, zucchini, cherry tomatoes, and red onion), chopped
- ❖ 1 teaspoon dried herbs (such as thyme, rosemary, or oregano)
- ❖ Salt and pepper, to taste
- ❖ ¼ cup chopped fresh parsley or cilantro
- ❖ ¼ cup crumbled feta cheese or goat cheese (optional)
- ❖ ¼ cup toasted nuts or seeds (such as almonds, walnuts, or pumpkin seeds) (optional)

For the Lemon-Herb Vinaigrette:

- ❖ ¼ cup extra virgin olive oil
- ❖ 2 tablespoons freshly squeezed lemon juice
- ❖ 1 tablespoon honey or maple syrup
- ❖ 1 teaspoon Dijon mustard
- ❖ 1 clove garlic, minced
- ❖ 1 teaspoon dried herbs (such as basil, parsley, or thyme)
- ❖ Salt and pepper, to taste

Procedures:

- ❖ Preheat the oven to 400°F (200°C). Line a baking sheet with parchment paper or aluminum foil for easy cleanup.
- ❖ In a medium saucepan, combine the quinoa and water or vegetable broth. Bring to a boil, then reduce the heat to low, cover, and simmer for 15-20 minutes, or until the quinoa is tender and the liquid is absorbed. Remove from heat and let it sit, covered, for 5 minutes. Fluff the quinoa with a fork and set aside.
- ❖ While the quinoa is cooking, spread the chopped vegetables in a single layer on the prepared baking sheet. Drizzle with olive oil and sprinkle with dried herbs, salt, and pepper. Toss to coat evenly.
- ❖ Roast the vegetables in the preheated oven for 20-25 minutes, or until they are tender and slightly caramelized, stirring halfway through cooking.
- ❖ In a small jar or bowl, whisk together the extra virgin olive oil, lemon juice, honey or maple syrup, Dijon mustard, minced garlic, dried herbs, salt, and pepper to make the lemon-herb vinaigrette.
- ❖ In a large mixing bowl, combine the cooked quinoa, roasted vegetables, chopped parsley or cilantro, and crumbled feta cheese or goat cheese (if using).
- ❖ Drizzle the lemon-herb vinaigrette over the quinoa and vegetable mixture, tossing gently to coat all the ingredients evenly.
- ❖ Sprinkle with toasted nuts or seeds for added crunch and flavor, if desired.
- ❖ Serve the quinoa salad warm, at room temperature, or chilled, according to your preference.

Nutritional Value (per serving):

- ❖ **Calories:** 320 kcal
- ❖ **Protein:** 8g
- ❖ **Fat:** 18g
- ❖ **Carbohydrates:** 35g
- ❖ **Fiber:** 6g
- ❖ **Sugar:** 5g

Cooking Tips:

- ❖ Use any combination of your favorite vegetables for roasting, such as bell peppers, zucchini, cherry tomatoes, red onion, broccoli, or cauliflower.
- ❖ To save time, you can use pre-cut or frozen vegetables for roasting. Just make sure to adjust the cooking time accordingly.
- ❖ Customize the salad with your favorite fresh herbs, cheese, and nuts or seeds for added flavor and texture.
- ❖ Make extra quinoa salad to enjoy as leftovers for lunch or dinner throughout the week. It's a convenient and nutritious option for meal prep.

Health Benefits:

- ❖ **High Protein:** Quinoa is a complete protein, containing all nine essential amino acids, making it an excellent plant-based protein source for vegetarians and vegans.

❖ **Nutrient-Dense:** Quinoa is rich in vitamins, minerals, and antioxidants, including magnesium, iron, zinc, and vitamin E, which support overall health and well-being.

❖ **Fiber-Rich:** Quinoa and vegetables provide dietary fiber, which aids in digestion, promotes satiety, and helps regulate blood sugar levels.

❖ **Heart-Healthy Fats:** Olive oil and nuts or seeds contribute heart-healthy monounsaturated and polyunsaturated fats, which may help lower cholesterol levels and reduce the risk of heart disease.

❖ **Antioxidant-Packed:** Vegetables and herbs are loaded with antioxidants, vitamins, and minerals, which help protect against oxidative stress, inflammation, and chronic disease.

This **Quinoa Salad with Roasted Vegetables** is a flavorful and nutritious dish that's perfect for lunch or dinner. With its hearty quinoa, vibrant roasted vegetables, and zesty lemon-herb vinaigrette, it's sure to satisfy your taste buds and nourish your body. Enjoy it as a standalone meal or serve it as a side dish alongside grilled chicken, fish, or tofu. However you choose to enjoy it, this quinoa salad is bound to become a favorite in your recipe repertoire!

Turkey and Avocado Wrap

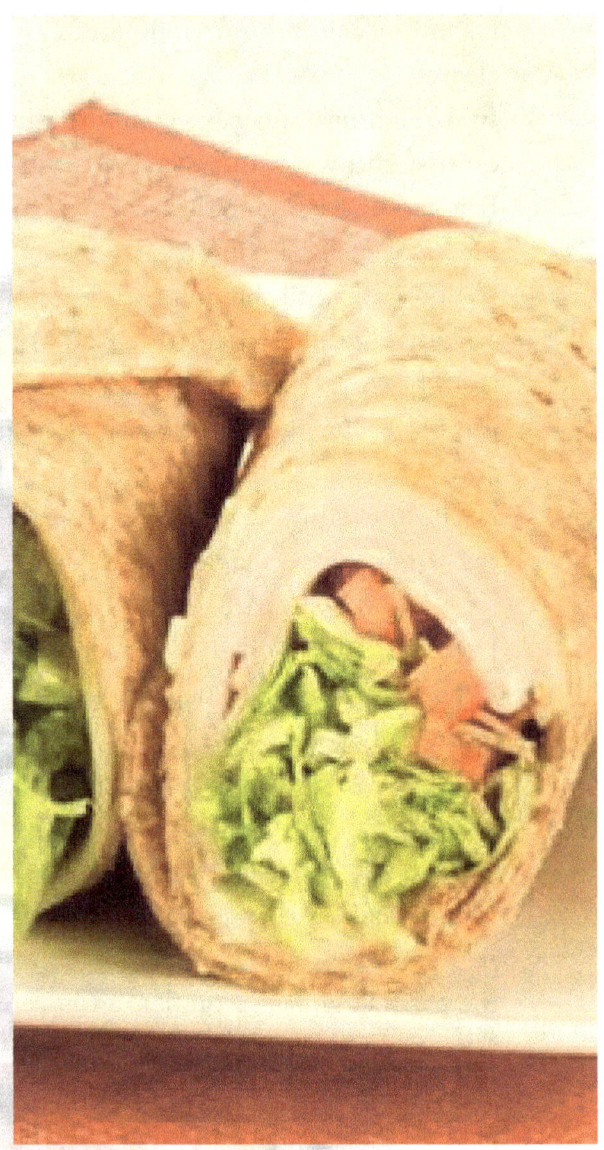

❖ **Preparation Time:** 10 minutes
❖ **Cooking Time:** 5 minutes (optional, for heating turkey)
❖ **Serving Unit:** Makes 2 wraps

Ingredients:

❖ 4 large whole wheat or spinach tortillas
❖ ½ pound sliced turkey breast
❖ 1 ripe avocado, thinly sliced

- ½ cup shredded lettuce or baby spinach leaves
- ¼ cup sliced red onion
- ¼ cup sliced cucumber
- ¼ cup shredded carrots
- ¼ cup hummus or Greek yogurt spread
- 2 tablespoons Dijon mustard or honey mustard
- Salt and pepper, to taste

Procedures:

- If desired, heat the sliced turkey breast in a skillet over medium heat for 1-2 minutes on each side, or until warmed through. Remove from heat and set aside.
- Lay out the tortillas on a clean work surface.
- Spread a thin layer of hummus or Greek yogurt spread evenly over each tortilla, leaving a border around the edges.
- Arrange the sliced turkey breast, avocado slices, shredded lettuce or spinach, sliced red onion, sliced cucumber, and shredded carrots in the center of each tortilla.
- Drizzle with Dijon mustard or honey mustard, and season with salt and pepper to taste.
- Fold in the sides of the tortilla, then roll it up tightly from the bottom to enclose the filling.
- Repeat with the remaining tortillas and filling ingredients.
- Slice each wrap in half diagonally before serving, if desired.

Nutritional Value (per serving, based on 1 wrap):

- **Calories:** 350 kcal
- **Protein:** 25g
- **Fat:** 15g
- **Carbohydrates:** 30g
- **Fiber:** 8g
- **Sugar:** 4g

Cooking Tips:

- Choose high-quality, thinly sliced turkey breast for the best flavor and texture in your wrap. You can use leftover roasted turkey or deli-style turkey slices.
- To add extra flavor, consider marinating the turkey breast in a simple marinade of olive oil, lemon juice, garlic, and herbs before cooking.
- If you prefer a warm wrap, you can heat the assembled wrap in a skillet over medium heat for 1-2 minutes on each side, or until lightly toasted and heated through.
- Customize the wrap with your favorite vegetables, spreads, and condiments. Try adding sliced tomatoes, bell peppers, sprouts, or pickles for added crunch and flavor.

Health Benefits:

- **Lean Protein:** Turkey breast is a lean source of protein, which is essential for muscle repair and growth, as well as overall health and vitality.

- ❖ **Healthy Fats:** Avocado provides heart-healthy monounsaturated fats, which may help lower cholesterol levels and reduce the risk of heart disease.
- ❖ **Fiber-Rich:** Whole wheat tortillas and vegetables provide dietary fiber, which aids in digestion, promotes satiety, and helps regulate blood sugar levels.
- ❖ **Vitamins and Minerals:** Vegetables like lettuce, spinach, red onion, cucumber, and carrots are packed with vitamins, minerals, and antioxidants, which support immune function and overall health.
- ❖ **Probiotics:** If using Greek yogurt spread instead of hummus, you'll benefit from the probiotics that support gut health and digestion.
- ❖ **Low-Calorie Option:** This turkey and avocado wrap is a nutritious and satisfying meal option that's lower in calories compared to heavier sandwiches or fast food options, making it a great choice for weight management.

This **Turkey and Avocado Wrap** is a delicious and nutritious meal that's perfect for a quick and satisfying lunch or dinner. With its combination of lean protein, healthy fats, fiber-rich vegetables, and flavorful condiments, it's sure to keep you fueled and satisfied throughout the day. Enjoy it at home.

Chicken Caesar Salad with Homemade Dressing

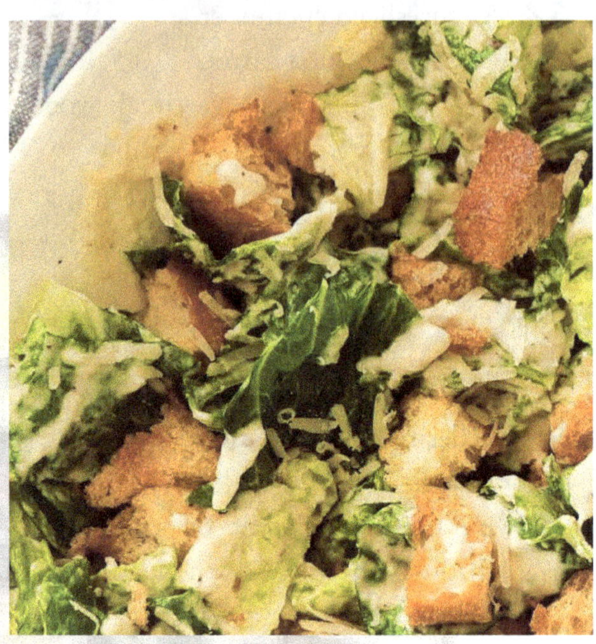

- ❖ **Preparation Time:** 20 minutes
- ❖ **Cooking Time:** 15 minutes
- ❖ **Serving Unit:** Makes 4 servings

Ingredients:

For the Chicken:

- ❖ 2 boneless, skinless chicken breasts
- ❖ 1 tablespoon olive oil
- ❖ 1 teaspoon garlic powder
- ❖ Salt and pepper, to taste

For the Caesar Dressing:

- ❖ ¼ cup mayonnaise
- ❖ 2 tablespoons grated Parmesan cheese
- ❖ 1 tablespoon lemon juice
- ❖ 1 teaspoon Dijon mustard
- ❖ 1 clove garlic, minced
- ❖ Salt and pepper, to taste

For the Salad:

* 1 large head of romaine lettuce, chopped
* 1 cup cherry tomatoes, halved
* ¼ cup grated Parmesan cheese
* ¼ cup croutons (optional)
* Anchovy fillets (optional, for garnish)
* Lemon wedges, for serving

Procedures:

Prepare the Chicken:

* Preheat the grill or grill pan over medium-high heat.
* Brush the chicken breasts with olive oil and season with garlic powder, salt, and pepper.
* Grill the chicken for 6-7 minutes on each side, or until cooked through and no longer pink in the center. Remove from heat and let it rest for a few minutes before slicing.

Make the Caesar Dressing:

* In a small bowl, whisk together the mayonnaise, grated Parmesan cheese, lemon juice, Dijon mustard, minced garlic, salt, and pepper until smooth and well combined. Adjust the seasoning to taste.

Assemble the Salad:

* In a large salad bowl, combine the chopped romaine lettuce and halved cherry tomatoes.
* Add the sliced grilled chicken on top of the lettuce and tomatoes.

* Drizzle the Caesar dressing over the salad, tossing gently to coat all the ingredients evenly.
* Sprinkle with grated Parmesan cheese and croutons, if using.
* Garnish with anchovy fillets, if desired.
* Serve immediately, with lemon wedges on the side.

Nutritional Value (per serving):

* **Calories:** 320 kcal
* **Protein:** 30g
* **Fat:** 18g
* **Carbohydrates:** 10g
* **Fiber:** 3g
* **Sugar:** 3g

Cooking Tips:

* For added flavor, marinate the chicken breasts in the Caesar dressing for at least 30 minutes before grilling. This will infuse the chicken with extra flavor and keep it moist and tender.
* Make sure to preheat your grill or grill pan before adding the chicken to ensure even cooking and beautiful grill marks.
* If you prefer, you can substitute the grilled chicken with leftover rotisserie chicken or cooked shrimp for a quicker and easier option.
* To make homemade croutons, toss cubed bread with olive oil, garlic powder, and dried herbs such as oregano or thyme. Bake in a preheated oven at 375°F (190°C) for 10-15 minutes, or until golden and crispy.

Health Benefits:

- ❖ **Lean Protein:** Chicken breast is a lean source of protein, essential for muscle repair and growth, as well as overall health and vitality.
- ❖ **Leafy Greens:** Romaine lettuce is rich in vitamins, minerals, and antioxidants, including vitamins A, C, and K, which support immune function and promote healthy skin and vision.
- ❖ **Omega-3 Fatty Acids:** Anchovy fillets are a source of omega-3 fatty acids, which have anti-inflammatory properties and are beneficial for heart health and brain function.
- ❖ **Healthy Fats:** Parmesan cheese provides calcium and protein, while mayonnaise and olive oil contribute heart-healthy monounsaturated fats.
- ❖ **Antioxidants:** Cherry tomatoes are packed with antioxidants, including vitamin C and lycopene, which help protect against oxidative stress and inflammation.

This **Chicken Caesar Salad with Homemade Dressing** is a classic and satisfying meal that's perfect for lunch or dinner. With its crisp romaine lettuce, juicy cherry tomatoes, tender grilled chicken, and creamy homemade Caesar dressing, it's sure to please your taste buds and nourish your body. Enjoy it as a standalone meal or serve it alongside crusty bread or a cup of soup for a complete and satisfying dining experience!

Black Bean and Corn Stuffed Sweet Potatoes

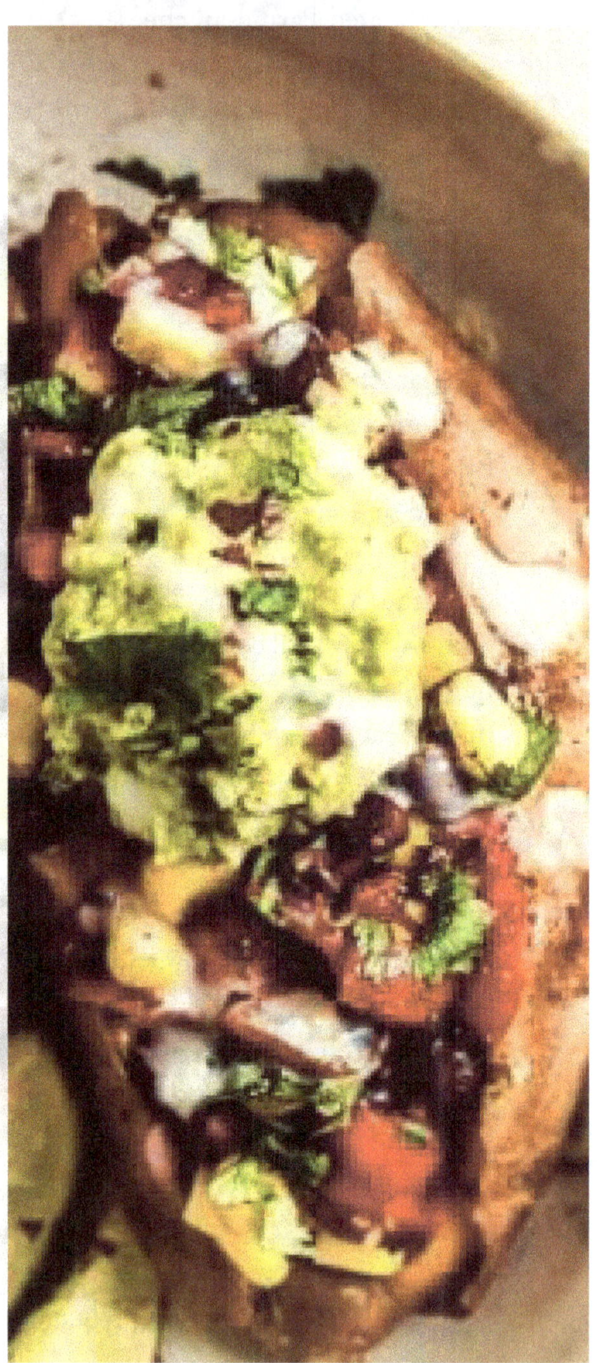

- ❖ **Preparation Time:** 15 minutes
- ❖ **Cooking Time:** 45 minutes
- ❖ **Serving Unit:** Makes 4 servings

Ingredients:

For the Stuffed Sweet Potatoes:

- ❖ 4 medium sweet potatoes
- ❖ 1 tablespoon olive oil
- ❖ 1 small onion, diced
- ❖ 2 cloves garlic, minced
- ❖ 1 teaspoon ground cumin
- ❖ 1 teaspoon chili powder
- ❖ ½ teaspoon smoked paprika
- ❖ 1 (15-ounce) can black beans, drained and rinsed
- ❖ 1 cup frozen corn kernels, thawed
- ❖ Salt and pepper, to taste
- ❖ Chopped fresh cilantro or parsley, for garnish

For the Homemade Dressing:

- ❖ ¼ cup Greek yogurt
- ❖ 2 tablespoons lime juice
- ❖ 1 tablespoon honey or maple syrup
- ❖ 1 tablespoon olive oil
- ❖ 1 clove garlic, minced
- ❖ Salt and pepper, to taste

Procedures:

Prepare the Sweet Potatoes:

- ❖ Preheat the oven to 400°F (200°C). Line a baking sheet with parchment paper.
- ❖ Wash the sweet potatoes and pierce them several times with a fork. Place them on the prepared baking sheet.
- ❖ Bake the sweet potatoes for 40-45 minutes, or until tender when pierced with a fork.

Make the Black Bean and Corn Filling:

- ❖ In a large skillet, heat the olive oil over medium heat. Add the diced onion and cook until softened, about 3-4 minutes.
- ❖ Add the minced garlic, ground cumin, chili powder, and smoked paprika to the skillet. Cook for an additional 1-2 minutes, until fragrant.
- ❖ Stir in the black beans and corn kernels, and cook for 3-4 minutes, until heated through. Season with salt and pepper to taste.
- ❖ Remove the skillet from heat and set aside.

Prepare the Homemade Dressing:

- ❖ In a small bowl, whisk together the Greek yogurt, lime juice, honey or maple syrup, olive oil, minced garlic, salt, and pepper until smooth and well combined. Adjust the seasoning to taste.

Assemble the Stuffed Sweet Potatoes:

- ❖ Once the sweet potatoes are cooked and cool enough to handle, slice them open lengthwise and fluff the flesh with a fork.
- ❖ Spoon the black bean and corn filling into the sweet potatoes, dividing it evenly among them.
- ❖ Drizzle each stuffed sweet potato with the homemade dressing.
- ❖ Garnish with chopped fresh cilantro or parsley.

Nutritional Value (per serving):

- ❖ **Calories:** 320 kcal
- ❖ **Protein:** 10g
- ❖ **Fat:** 8g
- ❖ **Carbohydrates:** 55g
- ❖ **Fiber:** 10g
- ❖ **Sugar:** 12g

Cooking Tips:

- ❖ To speed up the cooking process, you can microwave the sweet potatoes instead of baking them. Simply pierce them with a fork, place them on a microwave-safe plate, and microwave on high for 8-10 minutes, or until tender.
- ❖ Customize the filling with your favorite spices and herbs. Add a dash of hot sauce or chopped jalapeños for extra heat, or sprinkle with ground coriander or smoked paprika for additional flavor.
- ❖ For a creamier filling, mash some of the sweet potato flesh with the black bean and corn mixture before stuffing the potatoes.
- ❖ Make extra dressing and store it in an airtight container in the refrigerator for up to one week. It's delicious drizzled over salads, grilled vegetables, or as a dip for raw veggies.

Health Benefits:

- ❖ **High in Fiber:** Sweet potatoes, black beans, and corn are rich in dietary fiber, which aids in digestion, promotes satiety, and helps regulate blood sugar levels.
- ❖ **Plant-Based Protein:** Black beans provide plant-based protein, essential for muscle repair and growth, as well as overall health and vitality.
- ❖ **Vitamins and Minerals:** Sweet potatoes are a good source of vitamins A, C, and B-vitamins, as well as potassium and manganese, which support immune function and promote healthy skin and vision.
- ❖ **Probiotics:** Greek yogurt is a source of probiotics, which support gut health and digestion, as well as calcium and protein for bone health and muscle function.
- ❖ **Antioxidants:** Garlic, onions, and fresh herbs like cilantro and parsley are packed with antioxidants, vitamins, and minerals, which help protect against oxidative stress and inflammation.

These **Black Bean and Corn Stuffed Sweet Potatoes with Homemade Dressing** are a nutritious and satisfying meal option that's perfect for lunch or dinner. With their flavorful filling, creamy dressing, and tender sweet potato base, they're sure to please your taste buds and nourish your body. Enjoy them as a standalone meal or serve them alongside a fresh salad or soup for a complete and balanced dining experience!

Joey Ramsey

3

DINNER RECIPES

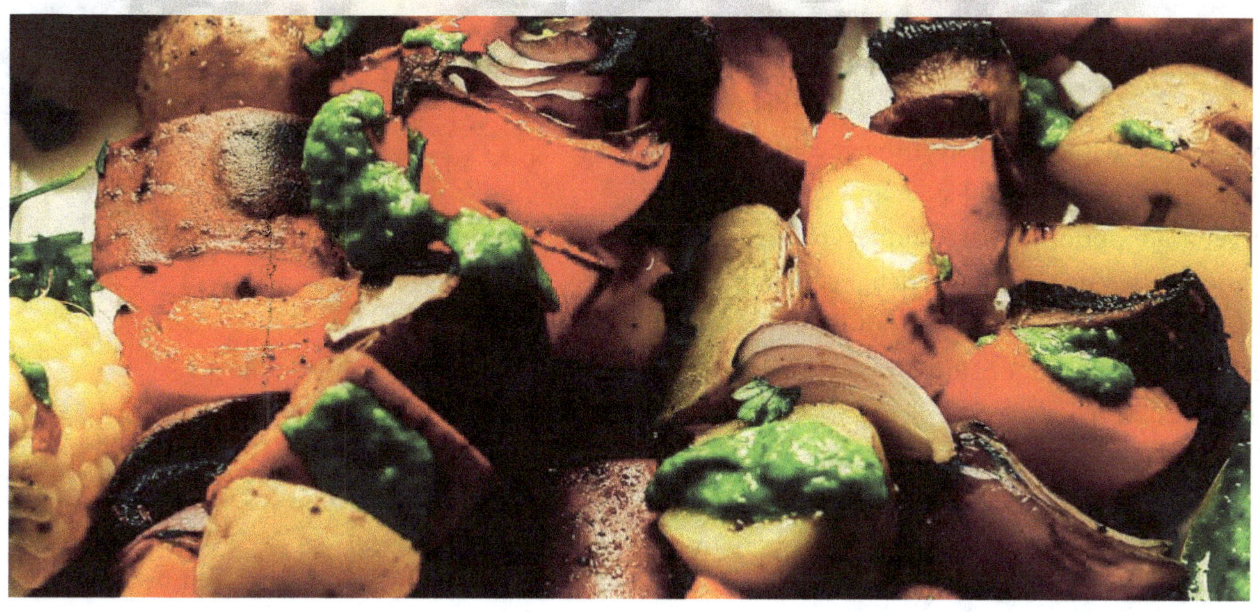

Nourishing Dinner Recipes for a Healthy Lifestyle

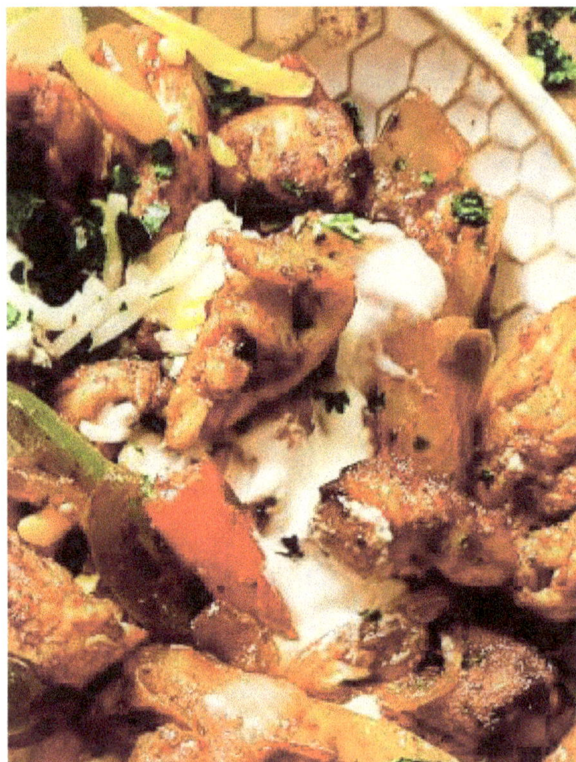

Lemon Garlic Roasted Salmon

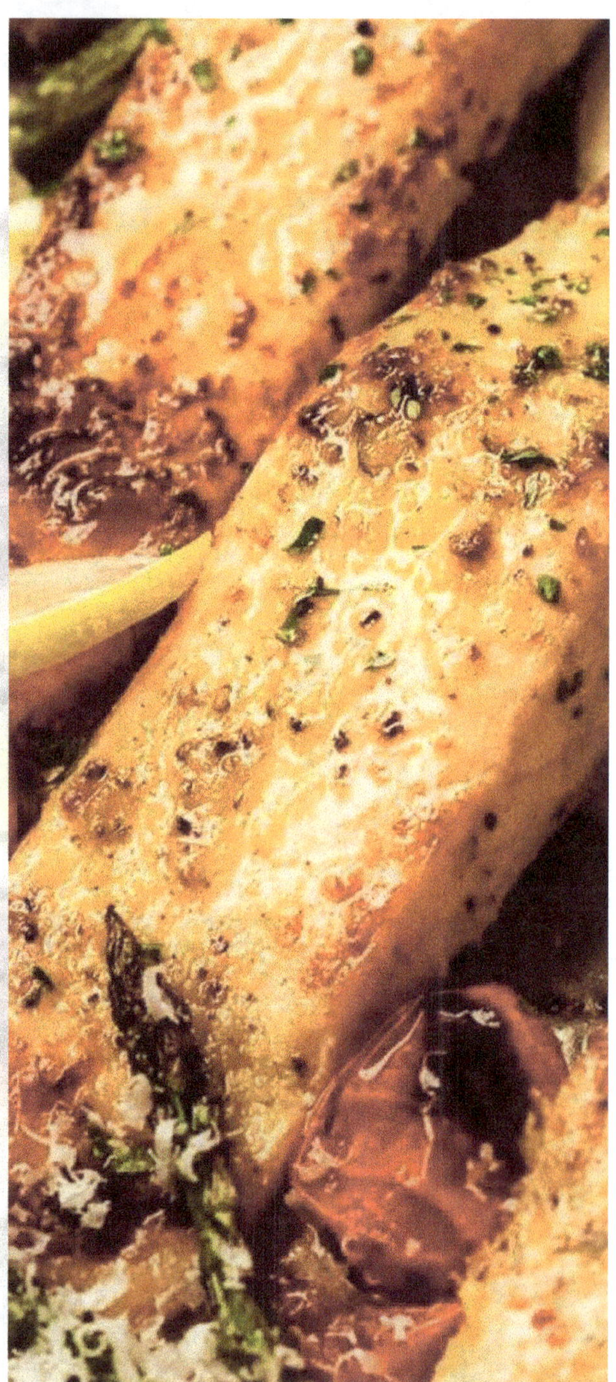

Welcome to the dinner section of the Galveston Diet Cookbook! Here, you'll find a diverse array of recipes to inspire your evening meals. From hearty mains to flavorful sides and wholesome vegetarian options, these dinner recipes are designed to nourish and delight. Whether you're cooking for a family dinner, entertaining guests, or simply enjoying a quiet night in, you'll discover plenty of delicious ideas to elevate your evening meals. So, let's explore the culinary possibilities and create memorable dinners that nourish both body and soul.

- ❖ **Preparation Time:** 10 minutes
- ❖ **Cooking Time:** 15-20 minutes
- ❖ **Serving Unit:** Makes 4 servings

Ingredients:

- 4 salmon fillets, skin-on or skinless, about 6 ounces each
- 2 tablespoons olive oil
- 4 cloves garlic, minced
- Zest of 1 lemon
- Juice of 1 lemon
- 1 teaspoon dried oregano
- 1 teaspoon dried thyme
- Salt and pepper, to taste
- Lemon slices, for garnish
- Chopped fresh parsley, for garnish

Procedures:

Preheat the Oven:

- Preheat the oven to 400°F (200°C). Line a baking sheet with parchment paper or aluminum foil for easy cleanup.
- Prepare the Salmon:
- Pat the salmon fillets dry with paper towels and place them on the prepared baking sheet.
- In a small bowl, whisk together the olive oil, minced garlic, lemon zest, lemon juice, dried oregano, dried thyme, salt, and pepper.

Marinate the Salmon:

- Drizzle the lemon garlic mixture over the salmon fillets, making sure to coat them evenly on all sides. Use your hands or a brush to spread the marinade over the salmon.

Roast the Salmon:

- Place the baking sheet in the preheated oven and roast the salmon for 15-20 minutes, or until the fish is opaque and flakes easily with a fork. Cooking time will vary depending on the thickness of the fillets.

Garnish and Serve:

- Once the salmon is cooked through, remove it from the oven and let it rest for a few minutes.
- Garnish the roasted salmon with lemon slices and chopped fresh parsley before serving.

Nutritional Value (per serving):

- **Calories:** 300 kcal
- **Protein:** 35g
- **Fat:** 16g
- **Carbohydrates:** 2g
- **Fiber:** 0g
- **Sugar:** 0g

Cooking Tips:

- Choose high-quality salmon fillets for the best flavor and texture. Look for fillets that are firm, moist, and brightly colored with no strong odor.
- If using skin-on salmon, you can place the fillets skin-side down on the baking sheet to prevent sticking. The skin will also help keep the salmon moist during roasting.
- For extra flavor, you can add sliced lemons or fresh herbs like rosemary or dill to the baking sheet before roasting.

❖ Avoid overcooking the salmon, as it can become dry and tough. Keep an eye on the fish and remove it from the oven as soon as it flakes easily with a fork.

Health Benefits:

❖ **Omega-3 Fatty Acids:** Salmon is rich in omega-3 fatty acids, which have been linked to numerous health benefits, including reduced inflammation, improved heart health, and enhanced brain function.

❖ **Lean Protein:** Salmon is a great source of high-quality protein, essential for muscle repair and growth, as well as overall health and vitality.

❖ **Antioxidants:** Garlic and lemon are packed with antioxidants, vitamins, and minerals, which help protect against oxidative stress and support immune function.

❖ **Heart Health:** The combination of omega-3 fatty acids and healthy fats from olive oil in this recipe may help lower cholesterol levels, reduce the risk of heart disease, and support cardiovascular health.

❖ **Low-Carb Option:** This lemon garlic roasted salmon is low in carbohydrates and sugar, making it suitable for low-carb and ketogenic diets.

Lemon Garlic Roasted Salmon is a simple yet elegant dish that's perfect for any occasion. With its vibrant flavors and tender, flaky texture, it's sure to impress your family and friends. Enjoy it as a centerpiece for a special dinner or as a quick and nutritious weeknight meal. Whether you're a seafood lover or looking to incorporate more heart-healthy omega-3s into your diet, this recipe is a delicious and satisfying choice!

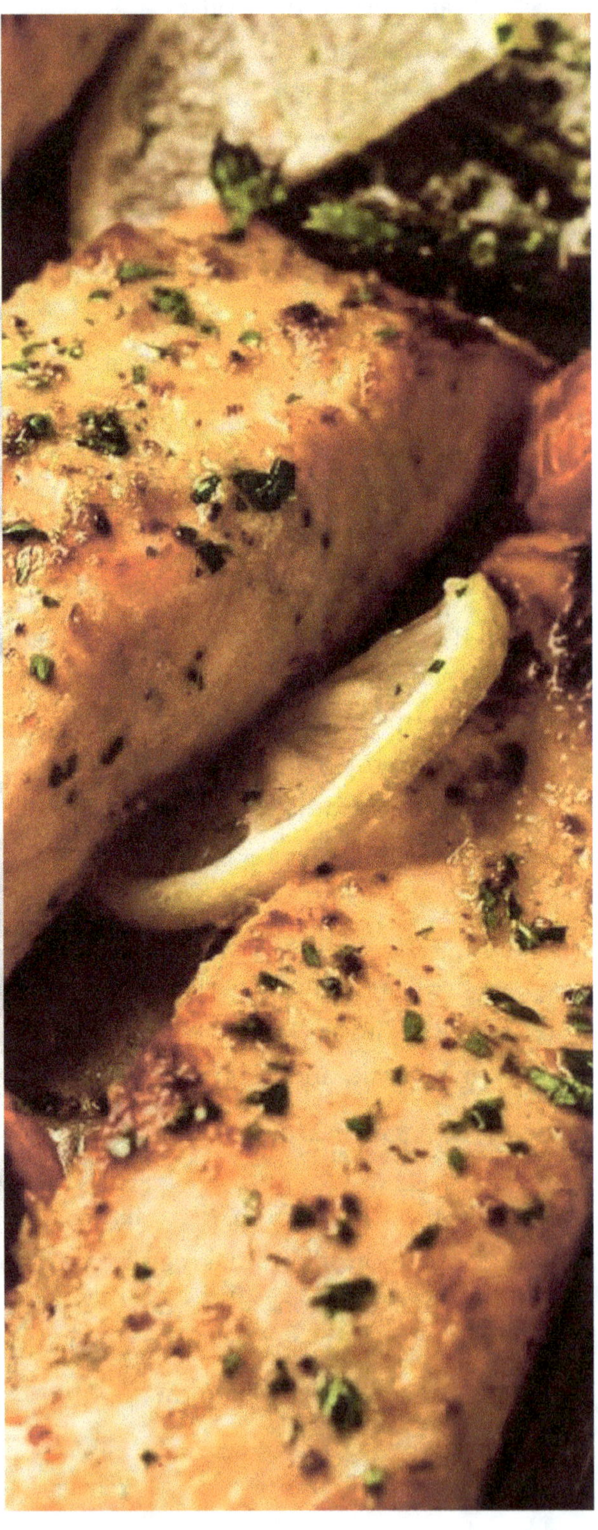

Chicken Fajita Bowl

- **Preparation Time:** 15 minutes
- **Cooking Time:** 20 minutes
- **Serving Unit:** Makes 4 servings

Ingredients:

For the Chicken Marinade:

- 1 pound boneless, skinless chicken breasts, thinly sliced
- 2 tablespoons olive oil
- 2 tablespoons lime juice
- 2 cloves garlic, minced
- 1 teaspoon chili powder
- 1 teaspoon ground cumin
- ½ teaspoon smoked paprika
- Salt and pepper, to taste

For the Fajita Bowl:

- 2 bell peppers (any color), thinly sliced
- 1 onion, thinly sliced
- 2 tablespoons olive oil
- Salt and pepper, to taste
- 4 cups cooked brown rice or cauliflower rice
- 1 cup canned black beans, drained and rinsed
- 1 avocado, sliced
- Fresh cilantro, for garnish
- Lime wedges, for serving
- **Optional toppings:** salsa, Greek yogurt or sour cream, shredded cheese

Procedures:

Marinate the Chicken:

- In a mixing bowl, combine the olive oil, lime juice, minced garlic, chili powder, ground cumin, smoked paprika, salt, and pepper to make the marinade.
- Add the thinly sliced chicken breasts to the marinade and toss until evenly coated. Cover and refrigerate for at least 30 minutes, or up to 4 hours.

Prepare the Vegetables:

- While the chicken is marinating, thinly slice the bell peppers and onion.
- In a large skillet, heat 2 tablespoons of olive oil over medium-high heat. Add the sliced peppers and onion to the skillet and sauté for 5-7 minutes, or until tender and slightly caramelized. Season with salt and pepper to taste. Remove from heat and set aside.

Cook the Chicken:

- In the same skillet, add the marinated chicken slices in a single layer. Cook for 6-8 minutes, stirring occasionally, until the chicken is cooked through and browned on all sides.

Assemble the Fajita Bowls:

- Divide the cooked rice evenly among serving bowls.
- Top each bowl with the cooked chicken, sautéed peppers and onions, black beans, and sliced avocado.
- Garnish with fresh cilantro and serve with lime wedges on the side.
- Optional: Add toppings such as salsa, Greek yogurt or sour cream, and

shredded cheese according to preference.

Nutritional Value (per serving):

- ❖ Calories: 450 kcal
- ❖ Protein: 30g
- ❖ Fat: 18g
- ❖ Carbohydrates: 45g
- ❖ Fiber: 10g
- ❖ Sugar: 3g

Cooking Tips:

- ❖ To save time, you can marinate the chicken overnight in the refrigerator, allowing the flavors to intensify and the chicken to become tenderer.
- ❖ If you prefer spicier fajitas, add a pinch of cayenne pepper or red pepper flakes to the marinade for an extra kick.
- ❖ Customize the fajita bowls with your favorite toppings and add-ons. Try adding diced tomatoes, shredded lettuce, sliced jalapeños, or guacamole for additional flavor and texture.
- ❖ For a low-carb option, substitute cauliflower rice for brown rice. Simply pulse cauliflower florets in a food processor until they resemble rice grains, then sauté in a skillet until tender.

Health Benefits:

- ❖ **Lean Protein:** Chicken is a lean source of protein, essential for muscle repair and growth, as well as overall health and vitality.
- ❖ **Fiber-Rich:** Brown rice and black beans provide dietary fiber, which aids in digestion, promotes satiety, and helps regulate blood sugar levels.
- ❖ **Antioxidants:** Bell peppers and onions are rich in vitamins, minerals, and antioxidants, including vitamins A and C, which help protect against oxidative stress and inflammation.
- ❖ **Healthy Fats:** Avocado provides heart-healthy monounsaturated fats, which may help lower cholesterol levels and reduce the risk of heart disease.
- ❖ **Versatile Nutrients:** Fajita bowls are packed with essential nutrients, including vitamins, minerals, and antioxidants, which support overall health and well-being.

Chicken Fajita Bowls are a delicious and nutritious meal option that's perfect for a quick and satisfying dinner. With their flavorful marinated chicken, sautéed peppers and onions, and hearty rice and bean base, they're sure to please the whole family. Enjoy them as a standalone meal or serve them alongside your favorite Mexican-inspired sides for a complete and balanced dining experience!

Cauliflower Fried Rice with Shrimp

- ❖ **Preparation Time:** 15 minutes
- ❖ **Cooking Time:** 15 minutes
- ❖ **Serving Unit:** Makes 4 servings

Ingredients:

For the Cauliflower Rice:

- ❖ 1 large head cauliflower, cut into florets
- ❖ 2 tablespoons olive oil
- ❖ 2 cloves garlic, minced
- ❖ 1 small onion, diced
- ❖ 2 carrots, diced
- ❖ 1 cup frozen peas, thawed
- ❖ 2 eggs, beaten
- ❖ 4 green onions, thinly sliced
- ❖ Salt and pepper, to taste

For the Shrimp:

- ❖ 1 pound shrimp, peeled and deveined
- ❖ 1 tablespoon soy sauce or tamari
- ❖ 1 tablespoon sesame oil
- ❖ 1 teaspoon grated ginger
- ❖ 2 cloves garlic, minced
- ❖ Salt and pepper, to taste
- ❖ **Optional garnishes:** chopped cilantro, sesame seeds, sliced green onions

Procedures:

Prepare the Cauliflower Rice:

- ❖ In a food processor, pulse the cauliflower florets until they resemble rice grains.

- ❖ Heat 1 tablespoon of olive oil in a large skillet or wok over medium heat. Add the minced garlic and diced onion, and cook until softened, about 2-3 minutes.
- ❖ Add the rice cauliflower and diced carrots to the skillet. Cook, stirring occasionally, until the cauliflower is tender, about 5-7 minutes.
- ❖ Stir in the thawed peas and cook for an additional 2-3 minutes.
- ❖ Push the cauliflower mixture to one side of the skillet and pour the beaten eggs into the empty space. Cook, stirring gently, until the eggs are scrambled and cooked through. Mix the scrambled eggs into the cauliflower rice.
- ❖ Season the cauliflower rice with salt and pepper to taste, and garnish with sliced green onions. Transfer the cauliflower rice to a serving dish and set aside.

Cook the Shrimp:

- ❖ In the same skillet or wok, heat the remaining tablespoon of olive oil over medium-high heat. Add the shrimp to the skillet in a single layer.
- ❖ Cook the shrimp for 2-3 minutes on each side, or until pink and opaque.
- ❖ Add the soy sauce or tamari, sesame oil, grated ginger, minced garlic, salt, and pepper to the skillet. Cook for an additional minute, stirring to coat the shrimp evenly with the sauce.

Assemble the Dish:

❖ Serve the cooked shrimp over the cauliflower fried rice.
❖ Garnish with chopped cilantro, sesame seeds, and sliced green onions, if desired.
❖ Serve hot and enjoy!

Nutritional Value (per serving):

❖ **Calories:** 250 kcal
❖ **Protein:** 25g
❖ **Fat:** 10g
❖ **Carbohydrates:** 15g
❖ **Fiber:** 6g
❖ **Sugar:** 6g

Cooking Tips:

❖ Make sure to thaw the frozen peas before adding them to the cauliflower rice to prevent the dish from becoming too watery.
❖ For a vegetarian option, you can omit the shrimp and add tofu or edamame instead.
❖ Customize the dish with your favorite vegetables and protein sources. Bell peppers, broccoli, mushrooms, and chicken are all delicious additions to cauliflower fried rice.
❖ To save time, you can use store-bought cauliflower rice instead of making it from scratch. Look for pre-riced cauliflower in the produce or freezer section of your grocery store.

Health Benefits:

❖ **Low-Carb Option:** Cauliflower rice is a low-carb alternative to traditional rice, making this dish suitable for low-carb and ketogenic diets.
❖ **High in Protein:** Shrimp is a lean source of protein, essential for muscle repair and growth, as well as overall health and vitality.
❖ **Packed with Vegetables:** Cauliflower fried rice is loaded with vegetables like cauliflower, carrots, peas, and green onions, providing essential vitamins, minerals, and antioxidants.
❖ **Heart-Healthy Fats:** Olive oil and sesame oil contribute heart-healthy monounsaturated and polyunsaturated fats, which may help lower cholesterol levels and reduce the risk of heart disease.
❖ **Gluten-Free:** This dish is naturally gluten-free, making it suitable for those with gluten sensitivities or celiac disease.

Cauliflower Fried Rice with Shrimp is a flavorful and nutritious dish that's perfect for a quick and satisfying dinner. With its tender shrimp, vibrant vegetables, and fragrant seasonings, it's sure to please your taste buds and nourish your body. Enjoy it as a standalone meal or serve it alongside your favorite Asian-inspired dishes for a complete and balanced dining experience!

Stuffed Bell Peppers with Ground Turkey

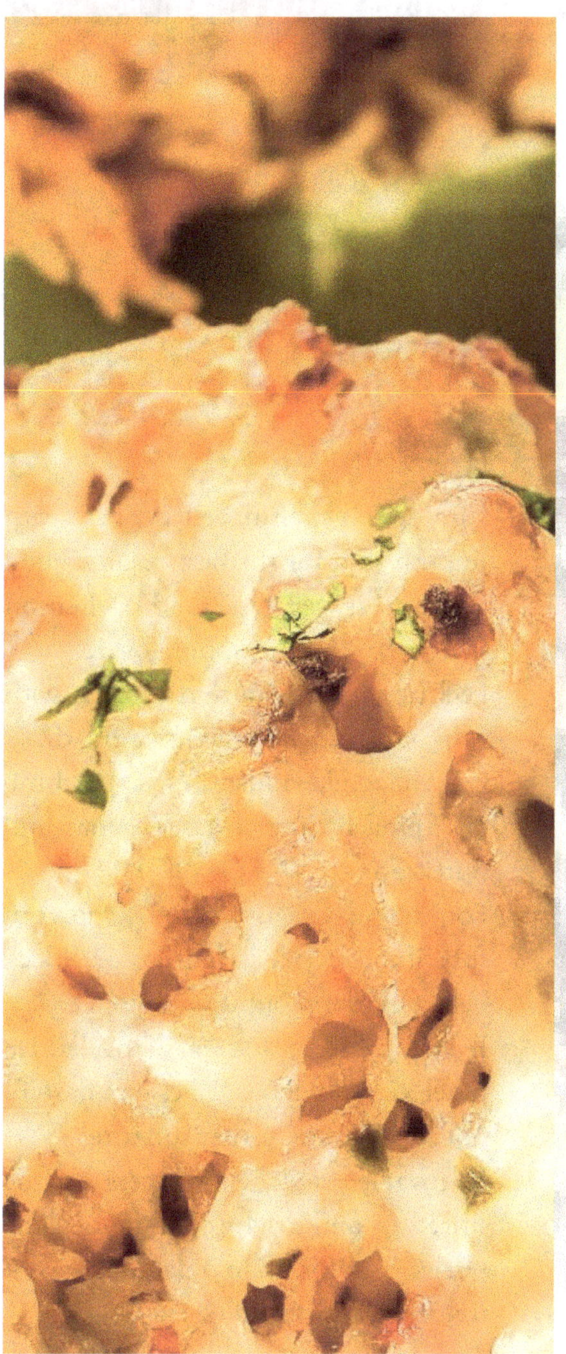

- ❖ **Preparation Time:** 20 minutes
- ❖ **Cooking Time:** 45 minutes
- ❖ **Serving Unit:** Makes 6 servings

Ingredients:

For the Stuffed Bell Peppers:

- ❖ 6 large bell peppers, any color
- ❖ 1 pound lean ground turkey
- ❖ 1 onion, diced
- ❖ 2 cloves garlic, minced
- ❖ 1 cup cooked quinoa or rice
- ❖ 1 cup diced tomatoes, fresh or canned
- ❖ 1 cup tomato sauce
- ❖ 1 teaspoon dried oregano
- ❖ 1 teaspoon dried basil
- ❖ Salt and pepper, to taste
- ❖ 1 cup shredded cheese (such as mozzarella or cheddar), optional

For garnish (optional):

- ❖ Chopped fresh parsley or cilantro
- ❖ Sliced green onions
- ❖ Sour cream or Greek yogurt

Procedures:

Preheat the Oven:

- ❖ Preheat the oven to 375°F (190°C). Grease a baking dish large enough to hold all the bell peppers.

Prepare the Bell Peppers:

- ❖ Slice the tops off the bell peppers and remove the seeds and membranes from the inside. Set aside.
- ❖ If needed, slice a thin layer off the bottom of each bell pepper to help them stand upright in the baking dish.

Prepare the Filling:

❖ In a large skillet, cook the ground turkey over medium heat until browned and cooked through, breaking it up with a spoon as it cooks.

❖ Add the diced onion and minced garlic to the skillet with the cooked turkey. Cook for 3-4 minutes, until the onion is soft and translucent.

❖ Stir in the cooked quinoa or rice, diced tomatoes, tomato sauce, dried oregano, dried basil, salt, and pepper. Cook for an additional 2-3 minutes, until heated through.

Stuff the Bell Peppers:

❖ Spoon the turkey and quinoa mixture evenly into each bell pepper, pressing down gently to pack the filling.

❖ If desired, sprinkle shredded cheese over the tops of the stuffed bell peppers.

❖ Bake the Stuffed Bell Peppers:

❖ Place the stuffed bell peppers in the greased baking dish. Cover the dish with aluminum foil.

❖ Bake in the preheated oven for 30-35 minutes, or until the bell peppers are tender.

❖ Remove the foil and bake for an additional 10 minutes, or until the cheese is melted and bubbly (if using).

Serve and Garnish:

❖ Remove the stuffed bell peppers from the oven and let them cool for a few minutes before serving.

❖ Garnish with chopped fresh parsley or cilantro, sliced green onions, and a dollop of sour cream or Greek yogurt, if desired.

Nutritional Value (per serving, without optional cheese):

❖ **Calories:** 250 kcal
❖ **Protein:** 20g
❖ **Fat:** 6g
❖ **Carbohydrates:** 30g
❖ **Fiber:** 6g
❖ **Sugar:** 6g

Cooking Tips:

❖ Choose large, firm bell peppers with smooth skin for the best results. Look for peppers that can stand upright on their own without tipping over.

❖ Feel free to customize the filling with your favorite ingredients. Add diced vegetables like mushrooms, zucchini, or spinach for extra flavor and nutrition.

❖ For a vegetarian option, you can substitute cooked lentils or black beans for the ground turkey.

❖ If you prefer a spicier filling, add a pinch of red pepper flakes or a dash of hot sauce to the turkey mixture.

❖ Leftover stuffed bell peppers can be stored in an airtight container in the refrigerator for up to 3 days. They also freeze well for longer storage.

Health Benefits:

❖ **Lean Protein:** Ground turkey is a lean source of protein, essential for muscle repair and growth, as well as overall health and vitality.

❖ **Whole Grains:** Quinoa or rice provides complex carbohydrates and dietary fiber, which help regulate blood sugar levels, promote satiety, and support digestive health.

❖ **Vitamins and Minerals:** Bell peppers are rich in vitamins A and C, as well as antioxidants, which help boost immune function and protect against oxidative stress.

❖ **Heart-Healthy:** This dish is low in saturated fat and cholesterol, making it a heart-healthy option that can help reduce the risk of heart disease.

❖ **Versatile Nutrients:** Stuffed bell peppers are a well-rounded meal that provides a balance of protein, carbohydrates, and fats, as well as essential vitamins, minerals, and antioxidants.

Stuffed Bell Peppers with Ground Turkey are a delicious and nutritious meal option that's perfect for a satisfying dinner. With their flavorful filling, tender bell peppers, and optional cheesy topping, they're sure to please the whole family. Enjoy them as a standalone meal or serve them alongside a fresh salad or steamed vegetables for a complete and balanced dining experience!

Grilled Veggie Skewers with Chimichurri Sauce

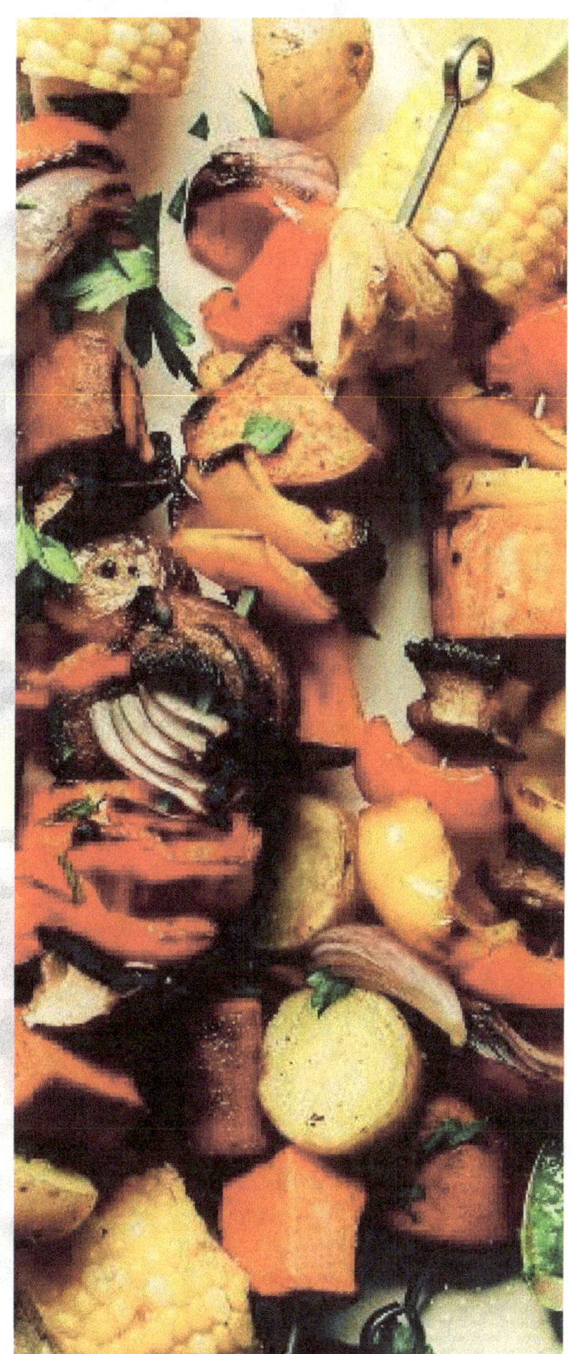

❖ **Preparation Time:** 20 minutes
❖ **Marinating Time:** 30 minutes
❖ **Cooking Time:** 10-15 minutes
❖ **Serving Unit:** Makes 4 servings

Ingredients:

For the Veggie Skewers:

- ❖ 2 bell peppers (any color), cut into chunks
- ❖ 1 large zucchini, sliced into rounds
- ❖ 1 large yellow squash, sliced into rounds
- ❖ 1 red onion, cut into chunks
- ❖ 8-10 cherry tomatoes
- ❖ 8-10 button mushrooms, cleaned
- ❖ Wooden skewers, soaked in water for at least 30 minutes

For the Chimichurri Sauce:

- ❖ 1 cup fresh parsley leaves, finely chopped
- ❖ ¼ cup fresh cilantro leaves, finely chopped
- ❖ 2 cloves garlic, minced
- ❖ ¼ cup red wine vinegar
- ❖ ½ cup olive oil
- ❖ 1 teaspoon dried oregano
- ❖ ½ teaspoon red pepper flakes (adjust to taste)
- ❖ Salt and pepper, to taste

Procedures:

Prepare the Chimichurri Sauce:

- ❖ In a small bowl, combine the finely chopped parsley, cilantro, minced garlic, red wine vinegar, olive oil, dried oregano, red pepper flakes, salt, and pepper. Stir well to combine. Adjust the seasoning to taste. Set aside to let the flavors meld while you prepare the veggie skewers.

Prepare the Veggie Skewers:

- ❖ Preheat the grill to medium-high heat.
- ❖ Thread the bell peppers, zucchini, yellow squash, red onion, cherry tomatoes, and mushrooms onto the soaked wooden skewers, alternating the vegetables as desired.

Grill the Veggie Skewers:

- ❖ Lightly brush the veggie skewers with olive oil and season with salt and pepper.
- ❖ Place the skewers on the preheated grill and cook for 10-15 minutes, turning occasionally, until the vegetables are tender and slightly charred.

Serve with Chimichurri Sauce:

- ❖ Once the veggie skewers are cooked through, remove them from the grill and transfer to a serving platter.
- ❖ Drizzle the chimichurri sauce over the grilled veggie skewers or serve it on the side as a dipping sauce.
- ❖ Garnish with additional fresh herbs, if desired.

Nutritional Value (per serving, without chimichurri sauce):

- ❖ **Calories:** 120 kcal
- ❖ **Protein:** 3g
- ❖ **Fat:** 7g
- ❖ **Carbohydrates:** 13g
- ❖ **Fiber:** 4g
- ❖ **Sugar:** 6g

Cooking Tips:

- ❖ Soak wooden skewers in water for at least 30 minutes before grilling to prevent them from burning.
- ❖ Cut the vegetables into uniform sizes to ensure even cooking on the grill.
- ❖ For extra flavor, you can brush the veggie skewers with a marinade before grilling. A simple mixture of olive oil, lemon juice, garlic, and herbs works well.
- ❖ Feel free to customize the veggie skewers with your favorite vegetables. Bell peppers, zucchini, yellow squash, red onion, cherry tomatoes, mushrooms, and eggplant are all great options.
- ❖ If using metal skewers, be sure to handle them with oven mitts or tongs as they can become very hot on the grill.

Health Benefits:

- ❖ Nutrient-Rich: Grilled vegetables are packed with vitamins, minerals, and antioxidants, which support overall health and well-being.
- ❖ Fiber: Vegetables are a good source of dietary fiber, which aids in digestion, promotes satiety, and helps regulate blood sugar levels.
- ❖ Heart-Healthy Fats: Olive oil in the chimichurri sauce provides heart-healthy monounsaturated fats, which may help lower cholesterol levels and reduce the risk of heart disease.

- ❖ Antioxidants: Fresh herbs like parsley and cilantro are rich in antioxidants, vitamins, and minerals, which help protect against oxidative stress and inflammation.
- ❖ Low-Calorie Option: Grilled veggie skewers are low in calories and fat, making them a healthy option for weight management and overall health.

Grilled Veggie Skewers with Chimichurri Sauce are a delicious and nutritious addition to any summer barbecue or outdoor gathering. With their vibrant colors, bold flavors, and tender-crisp texture, they're sure to be a hit with vegetarians and omnivores alike. Enjoy them as a standalone dish or serve them alongside grilled meats, seafood, or tofu for a complete and balanced meal!

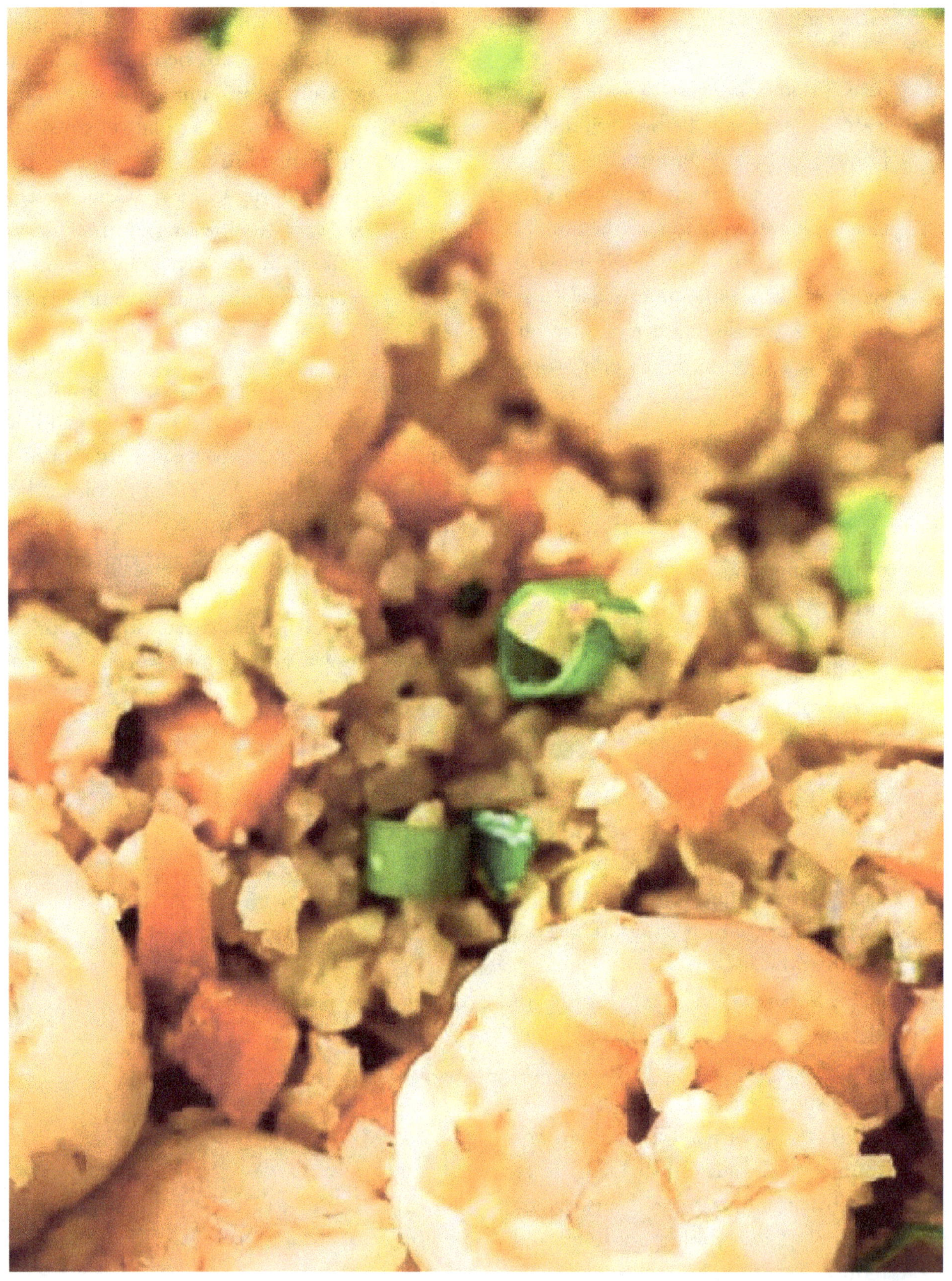

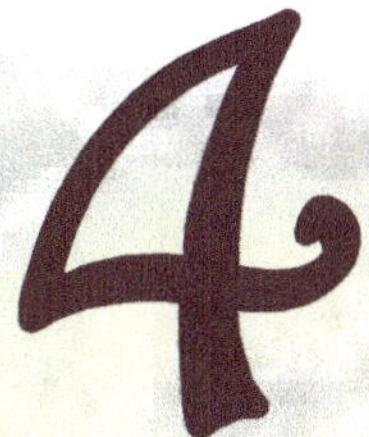

4

SNACK RECIPES

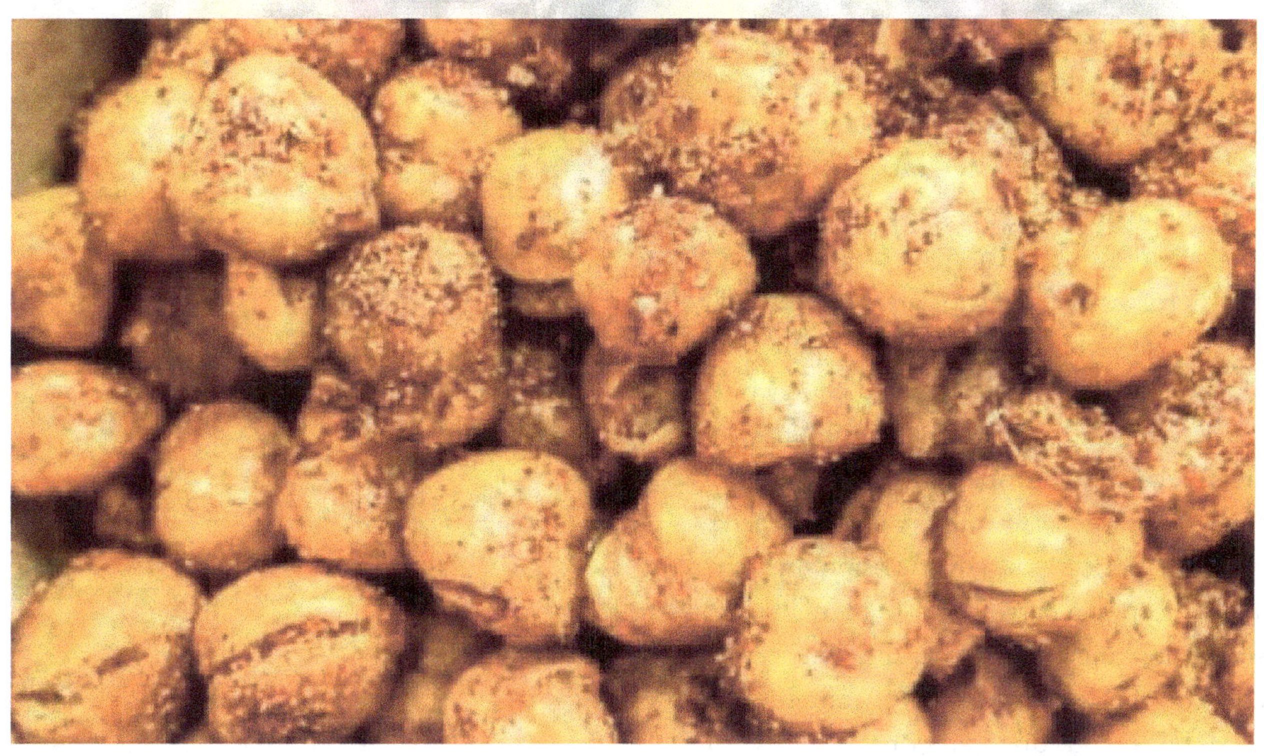

Joey Ramsey

Creative and Healthy Snacks Ideas

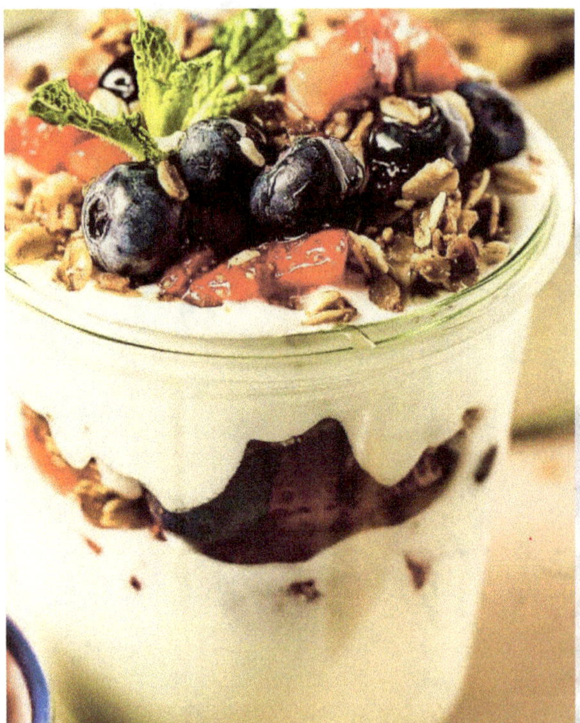

Guacamole with Homemade Baked Tortilla Chips

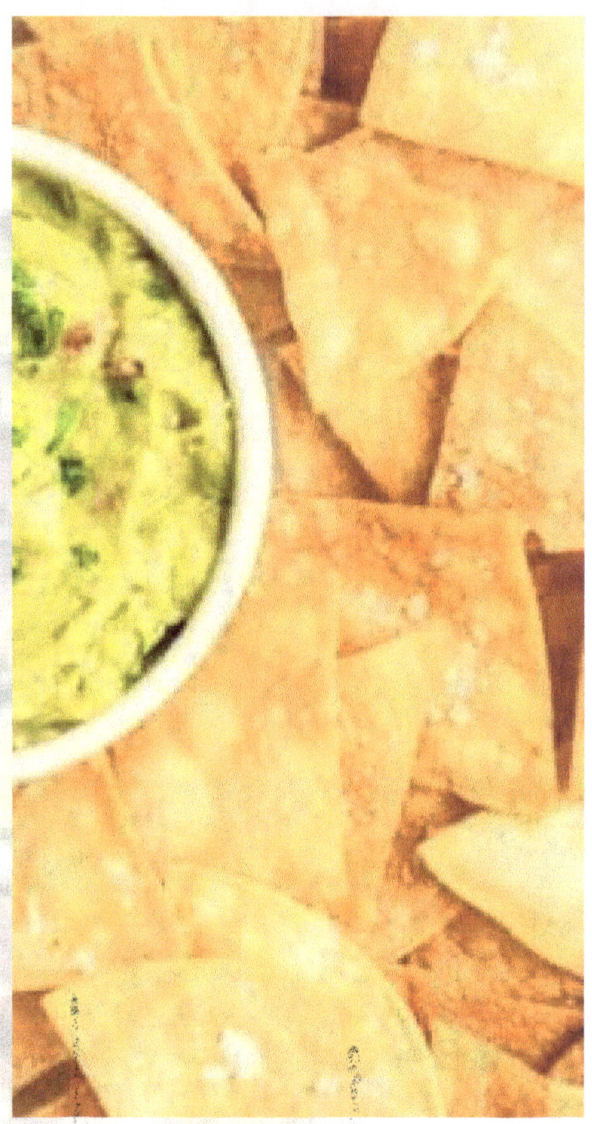

Snacks are the unsung heroes of the culinary world, providing delicious moments of satisfaction between meals, or as a pick-me-up during a busy day. Whether you're craving something savory, sweet, or somewhere in between, there's a snack recipe out there to satisfy every palate. From crunchy veggies with creamy dips to indulgent treats like homemade granola bars and energy bites, snack time offers endless possibilities for creativity and flavor exploration. In this section, we'll explore a variety of snack recipes that are perfect for any occasion, whether you're hosting a party, packing a lunchbox, or simply looking for a quick and tasty bite to enjoy on the go. So, get ready to tantalize your taste buds and discover your new favorite snack recipe!

❖ **Preparation Time (Guacamole):** 10 minutes

❖ **Preparation Time (Tortilla Chips):** 10 minutes

❖ **Cooking Time (Tortilla Chips):** 10-15 minutes

❖ **Serving Unit:** Makes about 2 cups of guacamole and a serving of tortilla chips

Ingredients:

For the Guacamole:

- 3 ripe avocados
- 1 small red onion, finely diced
- 1-2 tomatoes, diced
- 1 jalapeño pepper, seeded and minced (optional)
- ¼ cup chopped fresh cilantro
- Juice of 1-2 limes
- Salt and pepper, to taste

For the Homemade Baked Tortilla Chips:

- 6 corn tortillas
- 1 tablespoon olive oil
- Salt, to taste

Procedures:

Prepare the Guacamole:

- Cut the avocados in half and remove the pits. Scoop the avocado flesh into a medium-sized bowl.
- Mash the avocado with a fork until smooth or leave it slightly chunky, depending on your preference.
- Add the diced red onion, diced tomatoes, minced jalapeño pepper (if using), chopped cilantro, and lime juice to the mashed avocado. Mix well to combine.
- Season the guacamole with salt and pepper to taste. Adjust the seasoning and lime juice as needed. Cover the bowl with plastic wrap, pressing it directly onto the surface of the guacamole to prevent browning, and refrigerate until ready to serve.

- Prepare the Homemade Baked Tortilla Chips:
- Preheat the oven to 350°F (175°C). Line a baking sheet with parchment paper.
- Brush both sides of each corn tortilla with olive oil. Stack the tortillas and cut them into wedges using a sharp knife or pizza cutter.
- Arrange the tortilla wedges in a single layer on the prepared baking sheet. Sprinkle with salt to taste.
- Bake in the preheated oven for 10-15 minutes, or until the tortilla chips are golden brown and crisp. Keep an eye on them to prevent burning.
- Once baked, remove the tortilla chips from the oven and let them cool slightly before serving.

Nutritional Value (per serving, guacamole only):

- Calories: 120 kcal
- Protein: 2g
- Fat: 10g
- Carbohydrates: 8g
- Fiber: 5g
- Sugar: 1g

Cooking Tips:

- Choose ripe avocados for the best flavor and texture. They should yield slightly too gentle pressure when squeezed.
- To prevent the guacamole from browning, store it in an airtight container in the refrigerator and press

plastic wrap directly onto the surface before sealing.

❖ Customize the guacamole to suit your taste preferences by adjusting the amount of lime juice, cilantro, and jalapeño pepper.

❖ For extra flavor, you can add diced red bell pepper, minced garlic, or a pinch of cumin to the guacamole.

❖ For a spicier guacamole, leave the seeds in the jalapeño pepper or add a dash of hot sauce.

❖ Make sure to keep an eye on the tortilla chips while baking to prevent them from burning. They can go from golden brown to burn very quickly, so check them frequently.

Health Benefits:

❖ **Healthy Fats:** Avocados are rich in heart-healthy monounsaturated fats, which may help lower cholesterol levels and reduce the risk of heart disease.

❖ **Vitamins and Minerals:** Avocados are a good source of vitamins C, E, K, and B-6, as well as folate, potassium, and magnesium, which support overall health and well-being.

❖ **Antioxidants:** Tomatoes, onions, jalapeño peppers, and cilantro are all rich in antioxidants, vitamins, and minerals, which help protect against oxidative stress and inflammation.

❖ **Fiber:** Both avocados and corn tortillas are sources of dietary fiber, which aids in digestion, promotes satiety, and helps regulate blood sugar levels.

❖ **Low-Calorie Snack:** Homemade baked tortilla chips are a healthier alternative to store-bought chips, as they are lower in calories and fat, and free from artificial additives and preservatives.

Guacamole with Homemade Baked Tortilla Chips is a delicious and nutritious snack or appetizer that's perfect for parties, gatherings, or anytime you're craving a tasty treat. With its creamy avocado base, flavorful mix-ins, and crunchy tortilla chips, it's sure to be a hit with friends and family. Enjoy it as a standalone snack or serve it alongside your favorite Mexican-inspired dishes for a complete and satisfying meal!

Greek Yogurt Parfait with Fresh Fruit

- ❖ **Preparation Time:** 10 minutes
- ❖ **Serving Unit:** Makes 2 servings

Ingredients:

- ❖ 1 cup Greek yogurt (plain or flavored)
- ❖ 1 cup mixed fresh fruit (such as berries, sliced bananas, diced mango, or kiwi)
- ❖ ¼ cup granola or muesli
- ❖ 2 tablespoons honey or maple syrup (optional)
- ❖ Fresh mint leaves for garnish (optional)

Procedures:

Prepare the Ingredients:

- ❖ Wash and prepare the fresh fruit as needed. If using berries, rinse them under cold water and pat dry with a paper towel. Slice larger fruits like bananas, mangoes, or kiwis into bite-sized pieces.
- ❖ Assemble the Parfaits:
- ❖ In two serving glasses or bowls, layer the Greek yogurt, fresh fruit, and granola or muesli in alternating layers.
- ❖ Drizzle each parfait with honey or maple syrup, if desired, for added sweetness.
- ❖ Garnish with fresh mint leaves for a pop of color and extra freshness.

Nutritional Value (per serving):

- ❖ **Calories:** 200 kcal
- ❖ **Protein:** 15g
- ❖ **Fat:** 5g
- ❖ **Carbohydrates:** 30g
- ❖ **Fiber:** 5g
- ❖ **Sugar:** 20g

Cooking Tips:

- ❖ Use plain Greek yogurt for a tangy flavor, or choose flavored Greek yogurt for added sweetness. Greek yogurt is rich in protein and has a creamy texture that pairs well with fresh fruit.
- ❖ Experiment with different combinations of fresh fruit to create your own unique parfait. Berries, tropical fruits, and stone fruits all work well in this recipe.
- ❖ Choose a high-quality granola or muesli with whole grains, nuts, and seeds for added crunch and nutritional benefits.
- ❖ For extra flavor, you can sprinkle the granola with a pinch of cinnamon or nutmeg before layering it in the parfait.
- ❖ **Make-ahead tip:** You can prepare the parfaits in advance and store them in the refrigerator for up to 24 hours. Wait to add the granola until just before serving to keep it crunchy.

Health Benefits:

- ❖ **Protein-Rich:** Greek yogurt is an excellent source of protein, which helps keep you feeling full and satisfied between meals. It also provides essential amino acids for muscle repair and growth.

❖ **Rich in Vitamins and Minerals:** Fresh fruit is packed with vitamins, minerals, and antioxidants, which support overall health and well-being. Berries are particularly rich in vitamin C, while bananas provide potassium and mangoes offer vitamin A.

❖ **Fiber-Filled:** Both Greek yogurt and fresh fruit are good sources of dietary fiber, which promotes digestive health, regulates blood sugar levels, and helps prevent constipation.

❖ **Low in Added Sugar:** By sweetening the parfait with fresh fruit and a touch of honey or maple syrup, you can enjoy a naturally sweet treat without the need for excessive added sugar.

❖ **Versatile and Customizable:** This recipe is highly customizable, allowing you to tailor it to your taste preferences and dietary needs. You can swap out the fruit, yogurt, or granola for alternatives that suit your preferences or dietary restrictions.

Greek Yogurt Parfait with Fresh Fruit is a delicious and nutritious snack or breakfast option that's perfect for any time of day. With its creamy yogurt, sweet and juicy fruit, and crunchy granola, it's a satisfying treat that will leave you feeling energized and refreshed. Enjoy it as a quick and easy breakfast, a healthy snack between meals, or a light and refreshing dessert after dinner!

Spicy Roasted Chickpeas

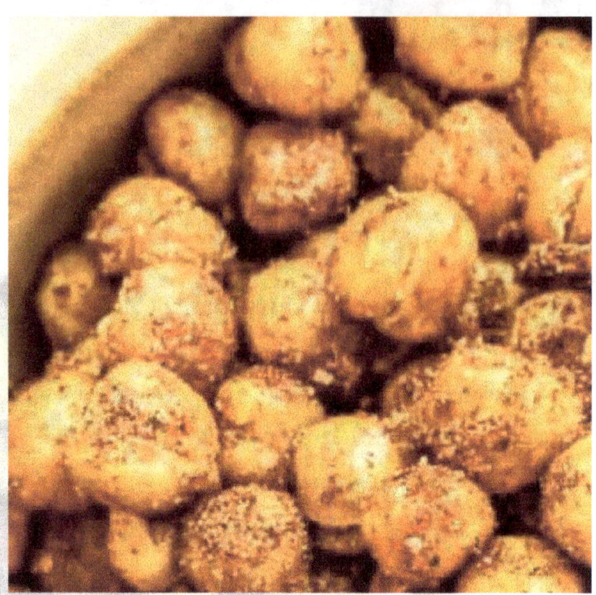

❖ **Preparation Time:** 10 minutes
❖ **Cooking Time:** 40 minutes
❖ **Serving Unit:** Makes about 2 cups

Ingredients:

❖ 2 cans (15 ounces each) chickpeas (garbanzo beans), drained and rinsed
❖ 2 tablespoons olive oil
❖ 1 teaspoon ground cumin
❖ 1 teaspoon paprika
❖ ½ teaspoon chili powder
❖ ¼ teaspoon cayenne pepper (adjust to taste for desired spiciness)
❖ ½ teaspoon garlic powder
❖ ½ teaspoon onion powder
❖ Salt, to taste
❖ Freshly ground black pepper, to taste

Procedures:

Preheat the Oven:

* Preheat your oven to 400°F (200°C). Line a large baking sheet with parchment paper or aluminum foil for easy cleanup.

Prepare the Chickpeas:

* Drain and rinse the chickpeas thoroughly under cold water. Pat them dry with a paper towel or kitchen towel to remove excess moisture.
* Spread the chickpeas out on the prepared baking sheet in a single layer.

Season the Chickpeas:

* Drizzle the chickpeas with olive oil, then sprinkle with ground cumin, paprika, chili powder, cayenne pepper, garlic powder, onion powder, salt, and freshly ground black pepper. Toss until the chickpeas are evenly coated with the seasonings.

Roast the Chickpeas:

* Place the baking sheet in the preheated oven and roast the chickpeas for 30-40 minutes, stirring halfway through, until they are crispy and golden brown.
* Keep an eye on the chickpeas towards the end of the cooking time to prevent them from burning. The exact cooking time may vary depending on your oven and the size of the chickpeas.

Cool and Serve:

* Once the chickpeas are roasted to your desired level of crispiness, remove them from the oven and let them cool slightly before serving.
* Enjoy the spicy roasted chickpeas as a crunchy and flavorful snack, or use them as a topping for salads, soups, or grain bowls.

Nutritional Value (per serving, about 1/4 cup):

* **Calories:** 120 kcal
* **Protein:** 5g
* **Fat:** 4g
* **Carbohydrates:** 16g
* **Fiber:** 5g
* **Sugar:** 1g

Cooking Tips:

* Make sure to thoroughly dry the chickpeas after rinsing them to ensure they get crispy during roasting. Excess moisture can prevent them from achieving the desired texture.
* Feel free to adjust the amount of spices according to your personal preference. If you prefer milder chickpeas, you can reduce the amount of cayenne pepper or omit it altogether.
* For added flavor, you can experiment with different spices and seasonings. Try adding smoked paprika, curry powder, or Italian seasoning for a unique twist.
* Store any leftovers in an airtight container at room temperature for up to 3 days. If the chickpeas lose their crispiness, you can reheat them in the

oven for a few minutes to revive their texture.

Health Benefits:

❖ High in Protein: Chickpeas are a good source of plant-based protein, which is essential for muscle repair and growth, as well as overall health and vitality.

❖ Rich in Fiber: Chickpeas are high in dietary fiber, which promotes digestive health, regulates blood sugar levels, and helps you feel full and satisfied.

❖ Heart-Healthy: Olive oil used for roasting the chickpeas provides heart-healthy monounsaturated fats, which may help lower cholesterol levels and reduce the risk of heart disease.

❖ Antioxidant-Rich: Spices like paprika, cumin, and chili powder are rich in antioxidants, which help protect against oxidative stress and inflammation in the body.

❖ Low in Calories: Spicy roasted chickpeas make a satisfying snack that's relatively low in calories compared to traditional snack foods like chips or pretzels. They're a great option for those looking to maintain or lose weight.

Spicy Roasted Chickpeas are a delicious and nutritious snack option that's perfect for satisfying your cravings for something crunchy and flavorful. With their crispy texture and bold spice blend, they're sure to become a favorite snack for any occasion. Enjoy them on their own as a healthy snack, or use them to add a crunchy topping to your favorite dishes for an extra burst of flavor and nutrition!

Cottage Cheese and Veggie Dip

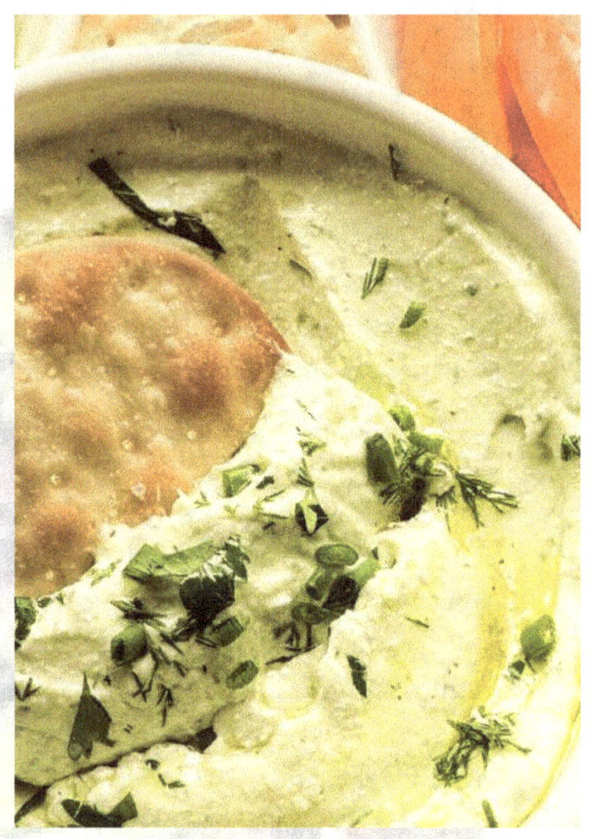

❖ **Preparation Time:** 10 minutes
❖ **Serving Unit:** Makes about 1 cup of dip

Ingredients:

❖ 1 cup cottage cheese (low-fat or full-fat)
❖ ½ cup finely chopped mixed vegetables (such as bell peppers, carrots, cucumber, celery, or cherry tomatoes)
❖ 2 tablespoons chopped fresh herbs (such as parsley, dill, chives, or basil)
❖ 1 clove garlic, minced
❖ 1 tablespoon lemon juice
❖ Salt and pepper, to taste

Procedures:

Prepare the Ingredients:

- ❖ Finely chop the mixed vegetables of your choice. You can use a combination of colorful bell peppers, crunchy carrots, refreshing cucumber, crisp celery, or juicy cherry tomatoes.
- ❖ Chop the fresh herbs finely. Popular options include parsley, dill, chives, or basil, but feel free to use any herbs you have on hand or prefer.
- ❖ Mince the garlic clove.

Make the Dip:

- ❖ In a blender or food processor, combine the cottage cheese, chopped vegetables, chopped herbs, minced garlic, and lemon juice.
- ❖ Blend or process the mixture until smooth and creamy, scraping down the sides of the bowl as needed.
- ❖ Taste the dip and season with salt and pepper to your liking. Adjust the seasoning and lemon juice as needed for desired flavor.

Serve:

- ❖ Transfer the cottage cheese and veggie dip to a serving bowl.
- ❖ Garnish with additional chopped herbs or a sprinkle of paprika for extra flavor and visual appeal.
- ❖ Serve the dip immediately with an assortment of fresh vegetables, crackers, or pita bread for dipping.

Nutritional Value (per serving, about 2 tablespoons):

- ❖ **Calories:** 40 kcal
- ❖ **Protein:** 5g
- ❖ **Fat:** 1g
- ❖ **Carbohydrates:** 3g
- ❖ **Fiber:** 0g
- ❖ **Sugar:** 2g

Cooking Tips:

- ❖ For a smoother dip, you can blend the cottage cheese mixture for a longer time until completely smooth. Alternatively, if you prefer a chunkier texture, you can pulse the mixture briefly to leave some small vegetable pieces intact.
- ❖ Customize the dip with your favorite vegetables and herbs. You can add diced red onion, minced jalapeño pepper, or grated radishes for extra flavor and heat.
- ❖ If you're short on time, you can use pre-chopped mixed vegetables from the grocery store to save on prep time.
- ❖ Make-ahead tip: This dip can be prepared in advance and stored in an airtight container in the refrigerator for up to 3 days. Stir well before serving, and add a splash of lemon juice if needed to freshen up the flavors.
- ❖ Experiment with different seasonings and flavorings to suit your taste preferences. Try adding a pinch of smoked paprika, cumin, or curry powder for a unique twist.

Health Benefits:

- ❖ Protein-Packed: Cottage cheese is a rich source of protein, which is essential for muscle repair and growth, as well as overall health and vitality.
- ❖ Nutrient-Rich: Mixed vegetables provide an array of vitamins, minerals, and antioxidants, which support immune function, promote healthy skin, and protect against chronic diseases.
- ❖ Low in Calories: This dip is relatively low in calories compared to traditional creamy dips made with sour cream or mayonnaise, making it a healthier option for snacking.
- ❖ Gut-Friendly: Cottage cheese contains probiotics, which are beneficial bacteria that support digestive health and promote a healthy gut microbiome.
- ❖ Versatile: This dip is versatile and can be enjoyed as a healthy snack, appetizer, or spread. Serve it with an assortment of fresh vegetables, crackers, pita bread, or whole grain chips for dipping.

Cottage Cheese and Veggie Dip is a creamy, flavorful, and nutritious dip that's perfect for snacking, entertaining, or adding a boost of protein and veggies to your meals. With its creamy cottage cheese base, crunchy mixed vegetables, and fresh herbs, it's a delicious and satisfying option that's sure to please the whole family. Enjoy it as a guilt-free dip for your favorite snacks or as a flavorful spread for sandwiches and wraps!

Almond Butter Energy Bites

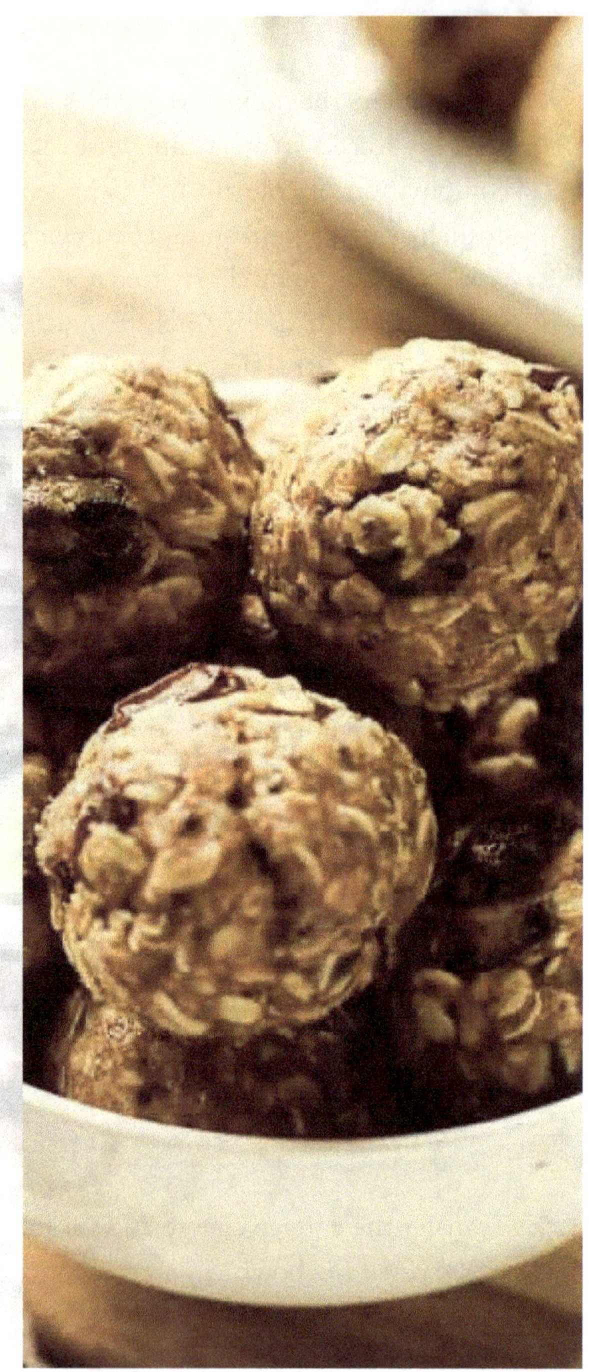

- ❖ **Preparation Time:** 15 minutes
- ❖ **Chilling Time:** 30 minutes
- ❖ **Serving Unit:** Makes about 20 energy bites

Ingredients:

- ❖ 1 cup rolled oats
- ❖ 1/2 cup almond butter (or any nut or seed butter of your choice)
- ❖ 1/4 cup honey or maple syrup
- ❖ 1/4 cup ground flaxseed or chia seeds
- ❖ 1/4 cup chopped almonds or other nuts (optional)
- ❖ 1 teaspoon vanilla extract
- ❖ 1/2 teaspoon ground cinnamon
- ❖ Pinch of salt
- ❖ Optional add-ins: dark chocolate chips, dried fruit, coconut flakes, protein powder

Procedures:

Mix the Ingredients:

- ❖ In a large mixing bowl, combine the rolled oats, almond butter, honey or maple syrup, ground flaxseed or chia seeds, chopped almonds (if using), vanilla extract, ground cinnamon, and a pinch of salt.
- ❖ Stir the mixture until well combined. If the mixture seems too dry, you can add a bit more almond butter or honey to help bind everything together.

Form the Energy Bites:

- ❖ Once the mixture is well combined, use your hands to roll it into small balls, about 1 inch in diameter. If the mixture is too sticky, you can bet your hands with water to prevent sticking.

Chill the Energy Bites:

- ❖ Place the rolled energy bites on a baking sheet lined with parchment paper or a plate. Transfer them to the refrigerator to chill for at least 30 minutes, or until firm.

Serve and Enjoy:

- ❖ Once the energy bites are chilled and firm, remove them from the refrigerator.
- ❖ Serve the almond butter energy bites immediately, or store them in an airtight container in the refrigerator for up to one week.

Nutritional Value (per energy bite):

- ❖ **Calories:** 80 kcal
- ❖ **Protein:** 2g
- ❖ **Fat:** 5g
- ❖ **Carbohydrates:** 7g
- ❖ **Fiber:** 1g
- ❖ **Sugar:** 3g

Cooking Tips:

- ❖ Customize the energy bites with your favorite add-ins. Dark chocolate chips, dried fruit (such as raisins, cranberries, or chopped apricots), coconut flakes, or protein powder are all great options for adding flavor and nutrition.
- ❖ If you prefer a sweeter energy bite, you can increase the amount of honey or maple syrup in the recipe. Alternatively, if you're watching your sugar intake, you can reduce or omit the sweetener altogether.

❖ Make sure to use natural almond butter without added sugars or oils for a healthier option. You can also use other nut or seed butters such as peanut butter, cashew butter, or sunflower seed butter.

❖ For extra texture and crunch, you can roll the energy bites in shredded coconut, chopped nuts, or cocoa powder before chilling.

❖ If you don't have ground flaxseed or chia seeds on hand, you can omit them from the recipe or substitute with additional rolled oats.

❖ These energy bites are great for meal prep and can be made in advance for a quick and convenient snack on the go. Store them in the refrigerator or freezer for longer shelf life.

Health Benefits:

❖ **Energy Boost:** Almond butter energy bites are packed with complex carbohydrates from rolled oats, which provide sustained energy to keep you fueled throughout the day.

❖ **Protein-Rich:** Almond butter and ground flaxseed or chia seeds are rich sources of plant-based protein, which is essential for muscle repair and growth, as well as overall health and vitality.

❖ **Healthy Fats:** Almond butter and almonds provide heart-healthy monounsaturated fats, which may help lower cholesterol levels and reduce the risk of heart disease when consumed as part of a balanced diet.

❖ **Fiber:** Rolled oats and flaxseed or chia seeds are high in dietary fiber, which promotes digestive health, regulates blood sugar levels, and helps you feel full and satisfied.

❖ **Nutrient-Dense:** Almond butter energy bites are packed with essential vitamins, minerals, and antioxidants from the nuts, seeds, and whole grains, which support overall health and well-being.

Almond Butter Energy Bites are a delicious and nutritious snack option that's perfect for busy days when you need a quick pick-me-up. With their balanced blend of protein, healthy fats, and carbohydrates, they provide a convenient and satisfying source of energy to keep you going throughout the day. Enjoy them as a pre-workout snack, afternoon pick-me-up, or healthy dessert alternative!

5

DESSERT RECIPES

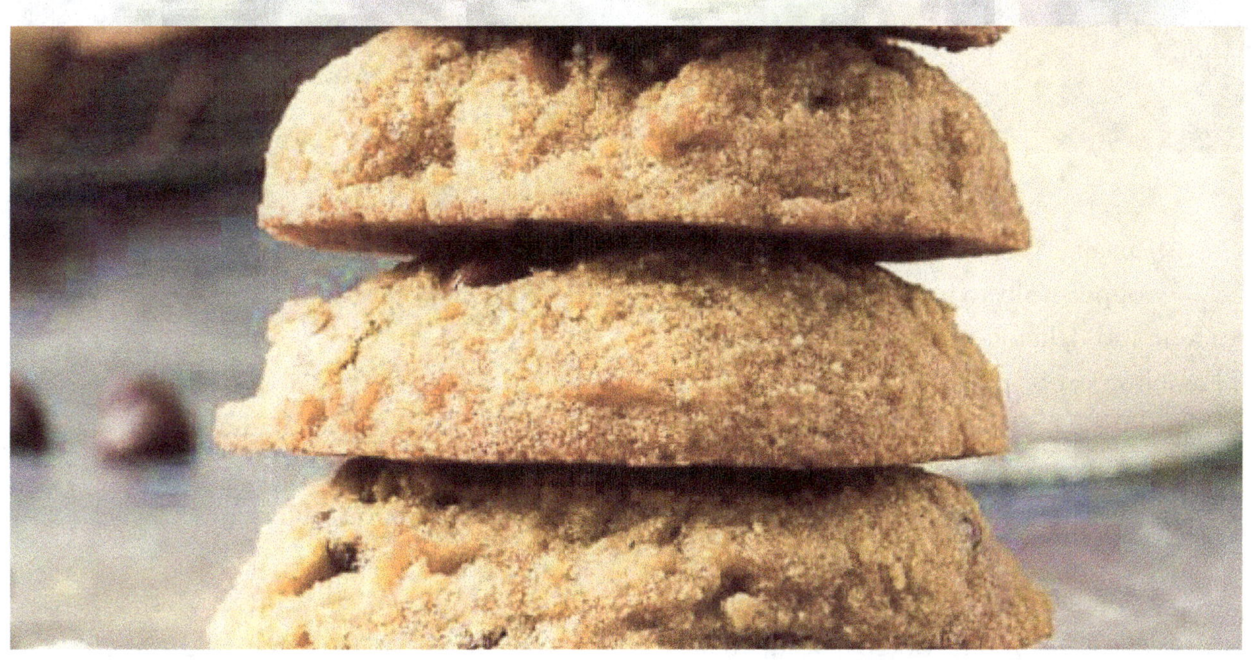

Indulge Your Sweet Tooth: Irresistible Dessert Recipes

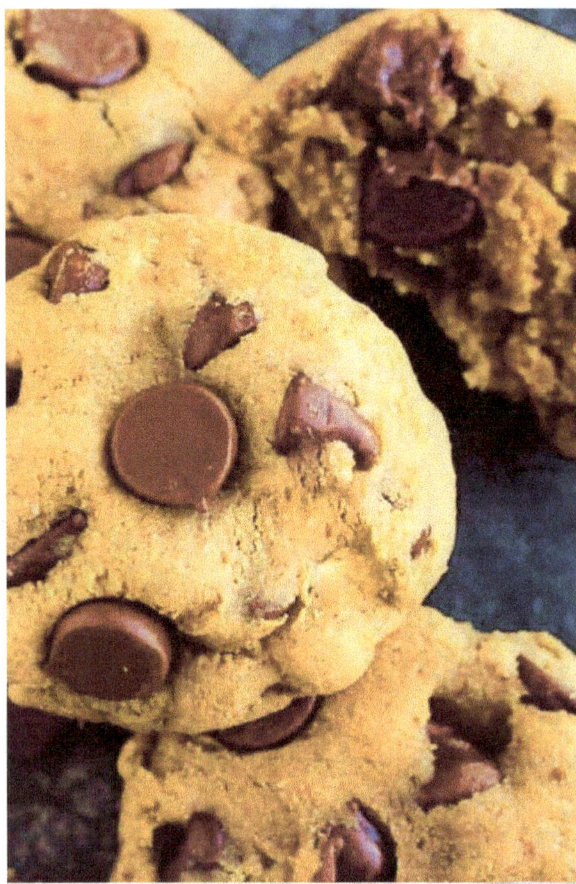

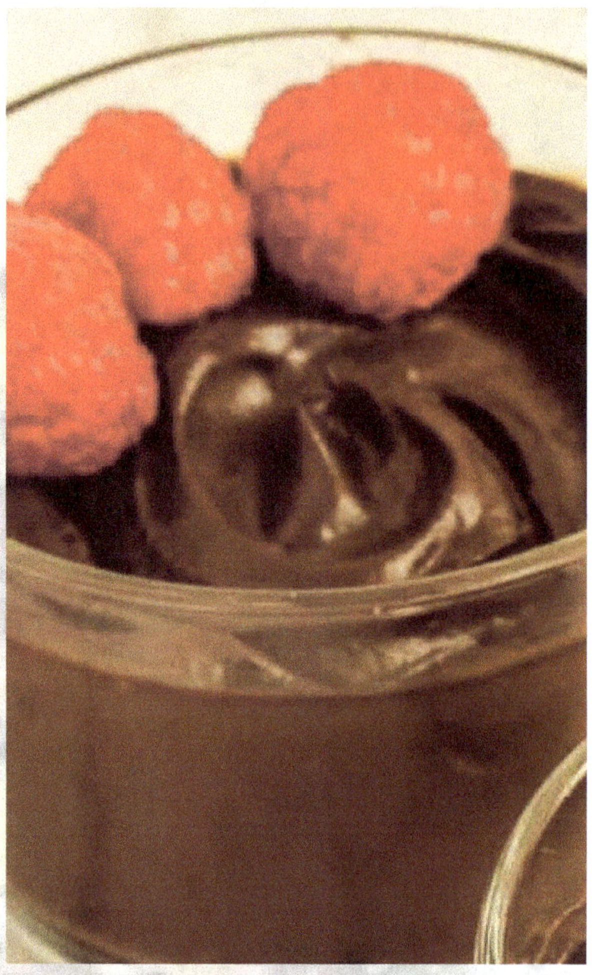

Dessert time is the sweetest part of any meal, offering a delightful opportunity to indulge in something decadent and delicious. In this section, you'll find a collection of irresistible dessert recipes that will satisfy your cravings and leave you wanting more. From classic favorites like chocolate chip cookies and creamy cheesecake to innovative treats like fruit-filled crumbles and silky pudding, there's something here to satisfy every sweet tooth. So go ahead, treat yourself to a little something sweet and savor the joy of dessert time!

❖ **Preparation Time:** 10 minutes
❖ **Chilling Time:** 1 hour
❖ **Serving Unit:** Makes about 4 servings

Ingredients:

❖ 2 ripe avocados
❖ ¼ cup unsweetened cocoa powder
❖ ¼ cup maple syrup or honey
❖ 1 teaspoon vanilla extract
❖ Pinch of salt
❖ **Optional toppings:** fresh berries, sliced bananas, chopped nuts, shaved chocolate

Procedures:

Prepare the Avocados:

- ❖ Cut the avocados in half and remove the pits. Scoop the avocado flesh into a blender or food processor.

Blend the Ingredients:

- ❖ Add the cocoa powder, maple syrup or honey, vanilla extract, and a pinch of salt to the blender or food processor with the avocado flesh.
- ❖ Blend the mixture until smooth and creamy, scraping down the sides of the blender or food processor as needed to ensure everything is well combined.

Chill the Mousse:

- ❖ Transfer the chocolate avocado mousse to serving glasses or bowls.
- ❖ Cover the glasses or bowls with plastic wrap or lids and refrigerate for at least 1 hour, or until the mousse is chilled and set.

Serve and Enjoy:

- ❖ Once the chocolate avocado mousse is chilled, remove it from the refrigerator.
- ❖ Garnish each serving with optional toppings such as fresh berries, sliced bananas, chopped nuts, or shaved chocolate, if desired.
- ❖ Serve the mousse immediately and enjoy the rich, creamy goodness!

Nutritional Value (per serving):

- ❖ **Calories:** 200 kcal
- ❖ **Protein:** 3g
- ❖ **Fat:** 15g
- ❖ **Carbohydrates:** 20g
- ❖ **Fiber:** 8g
- ❖ **Sugar:** 10g

Cooking Tips:

- ❖ Use ripe avocados for the best flavor and texture. They should yield slightly too gentle pressure when squeezed.
- ❖ Adjust the sweetness of the mousse to your taste preference by adding more or less maple syrup or honey.
- ❖ For a smoother mousse, blend the ingredients for a longer time until completely smooth. If you prefer a chunkier texture, you can pulse the mixture briefly to leave some avocado chunks intact.
- ❖ Get creative with toppings! Fresh berries, sliced bananas, chopped nuts, and shaved chocolate are all delicious options for adding extra flavor and texture to the mousse.
- ❖ Make sure to cover the mousse with plastic wrap or lids before refrigerating to prevent it from developing a skin on top.

Health Benefits:

- ❖ **Nutrient-Rich:** Avocados are packed with vitamins, minerals, and healthy fats, making them a nutritious addition to any dessert. They're rich in potassium, vitamin K, vitamin E, and folate, which support overall health and well-being.

❖ **Heart-Healthy Fats:** Avocados are a good source of monounsaturated fats, which may help lower cholesterol levels and reduce the risk of heart disease when consumed as part of a balanced diet.

❖ **Antioxidant-Rich:** Cocoa powder is high in antioxidants, which help protect against oxidative stress and inflammation in the body. It also contains flavonoids, which have been linked to various health benefits, including improved heart health and brain function.

❖ **Fiber-Filled:** Avocados and cocoa powder are both sources of dietary fiber, which promotes digestive health, regulates blood sugar levels, and helps you feel full and satisfied.

❖ **Lower in Added Sugar:** This chocolate avocado mousse is sweetened with natural sweeteners like maple syrup or honey, making it a healthier alternative to traditional desserts that are high in refined sugar.

Chocolate Avocado Mousse is a delicious and nutritious dessert option that's perfect for satisfying your sweet tooth without the guilt. With its rich, creamy texture and indulgent chocolate flavor, it's sure to become a new favorite in your dessert repertoire. Enjoy it as a decadent treat any time you're craving something sweet, and feel good knowing that you're nourishing your body with wholesome ingredients!

Berry Crisp with Oat Topping

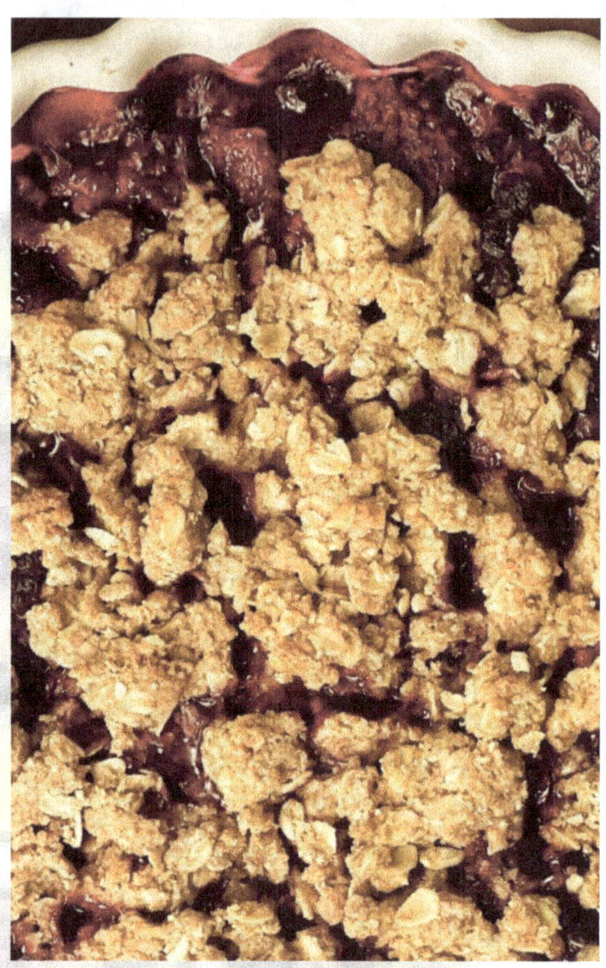

❖ **Preparation Time:** 15 minutes
❖ **Cooking Time:** 30-35 minutes
❖ **Serving Unit:** Makes about 6 servings

Ingredients:

For the Filling:

❖ 4 cups mixed berries (such as strawberries, blueberries, raspberries, and blackberries)
❖ ¼ cup granulated sugar
❖ 1 tablespoon cornstarch
❖ 1 tablespoon lemon juice

- ❖ Zest of 1 lemon
- ❖ ½ teaspoon vanilla extract

For the Topping:

- ❖ 1 cup old-fashioned rolled oats
- ❖ ½ cup all-purpose flour
- ❖ ¼ cup packed brown sugar
- ❖ ¼ cup granulated sugar
- ❖ ½ teaspoon ground cinnamon
- ❖ ¼ teaspoon salt
- ❖ ½ cup cold unsalted butter, cut into small cubes

Procedures:

Preheat the Oven:

- ❖ Preheat your oven to 350°F (175°C). Lightly grease a 9-inch square baking dish or a similar-sized oven-safe dish.

Prepare the Berry Filling:

- ❖ In a large mixing bowl, combine the mixed berries, granulated sugar, cornstarch, lemon juice, lemon zest, and vanilla extract. Toss the mixture gently until the berries are evenly coated with the sugar and cornstarch.

Make the Oat Topping:

- ❖ In a separate mixing bowl, combine the rolled oats, all-purpose flour, brown sugar, granulated sugar, ground cinnamon, and salt. Stir until well combined.
- ❖ Add the cold cubed butter to the oat mixture. Use your fingertips or a pastry cutter to incorporate the butter into the dry ingredients until the mixture resembles coarse crumbs.

Assemble and Bake the Crisp:

- ❖ Transfer the berry filling to the prepared baking dish, spreading it out evenly.
- ❖ Sprinkle the oat topping over the berry filling, covering it completely.
- ❖ Place the baking dish in the preheated oven and bake for 30 to 35 minutes, or until the berry filling is bubbling and the oat topping is golden brown and crisp.

Serve and Enjoy:

- ❖ Once the berry crisp is done baking, remove it from the oven and let it cool slightly before serving.
- ❖ Serve the warm berry crisp on its own or with a scoop of vanilla ice cream or a dollop of whipped cream, if desired.
- ❖ Enjoy the delicious combination of sweet, juicy berries and crunchy oat topping!

Nutritional Value (per serving):

- ❖ **Calories:** 300 kcal
- ❖ **Protein:** 3g
- ❖ **Fat:** 14g
- ❖ **Carbohydrates:** 43g
- ❖ **Fiber:** 5g
- ❖ **Sugar:** 25g

Cooking Tips:

- ❖ Use a variety of fresh or frozen berries for the filling to add color and flavor to the crisp. If using frozen berries, you may need to increase the baking time slightly.

❖ Adjust the sweetness of the berry filling according to your taste preference by adding more or less sugar. Sweeter berries may require less added sugar, while tart berries may need a bit more.

❖ For the oat topping, make sure the butter is cold and cut into small cubes to ensure a crumbly texture. You can also use a food processor to pulse the ingredients together if you prefer.

❖ Feel free to customize the oat topping by adding chopped nuts, coconut flakes, or spices like nutmeg or ginger for extra flavor and texture.

❖ Serve the berry crisp warm for the best flavor and texture. Leftovers can be stored in an airtight container in the refrigerator for up to 3 days and reheated in the oven or microwave before serving.

Health Benefits:

❖ **Antioxidant-Rich Berries:** Mixed berries are packed with antioxidants, vitamins, and minerals that help protect against oxidative stress and inflammation in the body. They're particularly rich in vitamin C, vitamin K, and fiber, which support overall health and well-being.

❖ **Whole Grain Oats:** The oat topping is made with old-fashioned rolled oats, which are a good source of complex carbohydrates, fiber, and protein.

Oats help regulate blood sugar levels, promote digestive health, and keep you feeling full and satisfied.

❖ **Heart-Healthy Fats:** The oat topping contains heart-healthy fats from the butter, which may help lower cholesterol levels and reduce the risk of heart disease when consumed as part of a balanced diet.

❖ **Lower in Added Sugar:** This berry crisp is sweetened with natural sugars from the berries and a small amount of granulated and brown sugar in the topping, making it a healthier alternative to traditional desserts that are high in refined sugar.

❖ **Fiber-Filled:** Berries and oats are both high in dietary fiber, which promotes digestive health, regulates blood sugar levels, and helps you feel full and satisfied. A diet rich in fiber may also help reduce the risk of chronic diseases such as heart disease, diabetes, and certain cancers.

Berry Crisp with Oat Topping is a delicious and wholesome dessert option that's perfect for showcasing the vibrant flavors of fresh or frozen berries. With its sweet and juicy berry filling and crisp, golden oat topping, it's sure to be a hit with family and friends alike. Enjoy it as a comforting treat on a warm summer evening or as a special dessert for any occasion!

Coconut Flour Chocolate Chip Cookies

- ❖ **Preparation Time:** 15 minutes
- ❖ **Cooking Time:** 10-12 minutes
- ❖ **Serving Unit:** Makes about 12 cookies

Ingredients:

- ❖ ½ cup coconut flour
- ❖ ¼ cup coconut oil, melted
- ❖ ¼ cup maple syrup or honey
- ❖ 2 eggs
- ❖ 1 teaspoon vanilla extract
- ❖ ¼ teaspoon baking soda
- ❖ Pinch of salt
- ❖ ½ cup dark chocolate chips

Procedures:

Preheat the Oven:

- ❖ Preheat your oven to 350°F (175°C). Line a baking sheet with parchment paper or silicone baking mat.

Mix Wet Ingredients:

- ❖ In a large mixing bowl, whisk together the melted coconut oil, maple syrup or honey, eggs, and vanilla extract until well combined.

Add Dry Ingredients:

- ❖ Add the coconut flour, baking soda, and a pinch of salt to the wet ingredients. Stir until a thick cookie dough forms. If the dough seems too dry, you can add a splash of milk or water to moisten it slightly.

Fold in Chocolate Chips:

- ❖ Gently fold in the dark chocolate chips until evenly distributed throughout the cookie dough.

Form Cookie Dough Balls:

- ❖ Use a spoon or cookie scoop to portion out the cookie dough and roll it into balls. Place the dough balls on the prepared baking sheet, spacing them a few inches apart to allow for spreading.

Bake the Cookies:

- ❖ Flatten each dough ball slightly with the palm of your hand to form a cookie shape.
- ❖ Place the baking sheet in the preheated oven and bake the cookies for 10 to 12 minutes, or until the edges are golden brown and the tops are set.
- ❖ Remove the cookies from the oven and let them cool on the baking sheet for a few minutes before transferring them to a wire rack to cool completely.

Nutritional Value (per cookie):

- ❖ **Calories:** 120 kcal
- ❖ **Protein:** 2g
- ❖ **Fat:** 8g
- ❖ **Carbohydrates:** 11g
- ❖ **Fiber:** 2g
- ❖ **Sugar:** 7g

Cooking Tips:

- ❖ Coconut flour tends to absorb more liquid than other flours, so it's important not to overdo it with the dry ingredients. If the dough seems too dry, you can add a bit more coconut oil or liquid sweetener to moisten it.
- ❖ Let the melted coconut oil cool slightly before adding it to the other wet ingredients to prevent the eggs from cooking.
- ❖ For extra flavor and texture, you can add chopped nuts, shredded coconut, or dried fruit to the cookie dough along with the chocolate chips.
- ❖ Keep an eye on the cookies towards the end of the baking time, as coconut flour cookies can go from golden brown to burn quickly.
- ❖ Allow the cookies to cool completely on a wire rack before storing them in an airtight container. They will continue to firm up as they cool.

Health Benefits:

- ❖ **Gluten-Free:** Coconut flour is naturally gluten-free, making these cookies suitable for those with gluten sensitivities or celiac disease.
- ❖ **Lower in Carbohydrates:** Coconut flour is lower in carbohydrates and higher in fiber compared to traditional wheat flour, which can help stabilize blood sugar levels and promote satiety.
- ❖ **Healthy Fats:** Coconut oil is a source of medium-chain triglycerides (MCTs), which are a type of healthy fat that can be easily digested and used for energy by the body.
- ❖ **Antioxidant-Rich Dark Chocolate:** Dark chocolate chips provide a rich source of antioxidants, particularly flavonoids, which have been linked to various health benefits, including improved heart health and cognitive function.
- ❖ **Moderate Sweetener:** Maple syrup or honey are used as natural sweeteners in this recipe, providing sweetness without the need for refined sugars. However, it's important to enjoy these cookies in moderation as they still contain added sugars.

Coconut Flour Chocolate Chip Cookies are a delicious and healthier alternative to traditional cookies, offering a chewy texture and rich chocolate flavor without the guilt. Made with wholesome ingredients like coconut flour, coconut oil, and dark chocolate chips, these cookies are perfect for satisfying your sweet tooth while still nourishing your body with nutritious ingredients. Enjoy them as a tasty treat any time you're craving something sweet, and feel good knowing that you're indulging in a healthier dessert option!

Frozen Yogurt Bark with Berries and Nuts

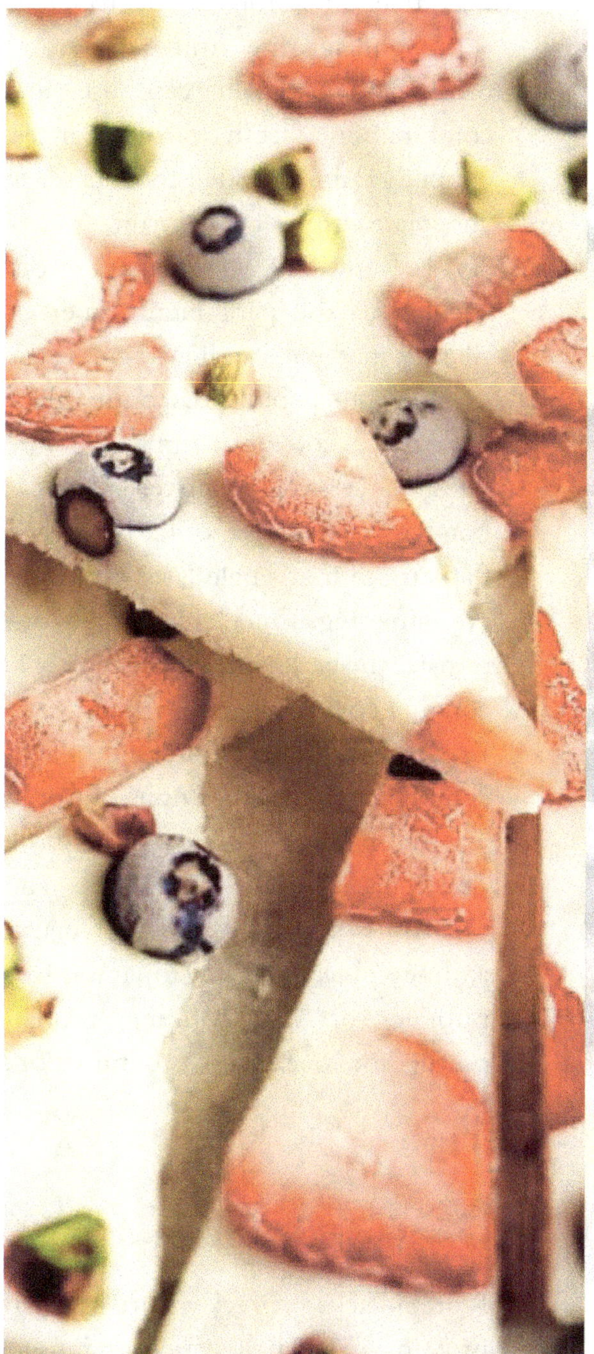

- ❖ **Preparation Time:** 10 minutes
- ❖ **Freezing Time:** 2-3 hours
- ❖ **Serving Unit:** Makes about 8 servings

Ingredients:

- ❖ 2 cups plain Greek yogurt
- ❖ 2 tablespoons honey or maple syrup
- ❖ 1 teaspoon vanilla extract
- ❖ 1 cup mixed berries (such as strawberries, blueberries, raspberries)
- ❖ ¼ cup chopped nuts (such as almonds, walnuts, or pecans)
- ❖ **Optional toppings:** shredded coconut, dark chocolate chips, dried fruit

Procedures:

Prepare the Yogurt Mixture:

- ❖ In a mixing bowl, combine the Greek yogurt, honey or maple syrup, and vanilla extract. Stir until smooth and well combined.

Spread the Yogurt Mixture:

- ❖ Line a baking sheet with parchment paper or a silicone baking mat.
- ❖ Pour the yogurt mixture onto the prepared baking sheet and use a spatula to spread it into an even layer, about 1/4 to 1/2 inch thick.

Add Toppings:

- ❖ Sprinkle the mixed berries and chopped nuts evenly over the yogurt layer, pressing them gently into the surface.
- ❖ If desired, add additional toppings such as shredded coconut, dark chocolate chips, or dried fruit for extra flavor and texture.

Freeze the Bark:

- ❖ Place the baking sheet in the freezer and freeze the yogurt bark for 2 to 3 hours, or until firm.

Break into Pieces:

- ❖ Once the yogurt bark is frozen solid, remove it from the freezer.
- ❖ Use your hands or a knife to break the bark into smaller pieces or cut it into squares.

Serve and Enjoy:

- ❖ Transfer the frozen yogurt bark pieces to a serving platter or container.
- ❖ Serve the bark immediately as a refreshing snack or dessert, or store any leftovers in an airtight container in the freezer for later enjoyment.

Nutritional Value (per serving):

- ❖ **Calories:** 90 kcal
- ❖ **Protein:** 6g
- ❖ **Fat:** 3g
- ❖ **Carbohydrates:** 11g
- ❖ **Fiber:** 2g
- ❖ **Sugar:** 8g

Cooking Tips:

- ❖ Use plain Greek yogurt for the base of the bark, as it has a thick and creamy texture that freezes well. You can use full-fat, low-fat, or non-fat Greek yogurt, depending on your preference.
- ❖ Sweeten the yogurt mixture to your taste preference with honey or maple syrup. Adjust the amount of sweetener based on the tartness of the yogurt and your personal preference for sweetness.
- ❖ Feel free to customize the toppings with your favorite fruits, nuts, and other add-ins. You can use any combination of fresh or frozen berries, chopped nuts, shredded coconut, dark chocolate chips, or dried fruit.
- ❖ To prevent the yogurt bark from sticking to the parchment paper or silicone mat, you can lightly grease the surface with a bit of coconut oil or non-stick cooking spray before spreading the yogurt mixture.
- ❖ For best results, freeze the bark on a flat surface in a single layer to ensure even freezing. Once frozen, you can transfer the bark pieces to a freezer-safe container for storage.
- ❖ Experiment with different flavor combinations and variations of frozen yogurt bark to suit your taste preferences and dietary needs. You can try using flavored Greek yogurt, adding spices like cinnamon or nutmeg, or incorporating protein powder for an extra boost of nutrition.

Health Benefits:

- ❖ Protein-Packed: Greek yogurt is rich in protein, which helps support muscle repair and growth, as well as overall health and vitality.
- ❖ Calcium-Rich: Yogurt is a good source of calcium, which is essential for

strong bones and teeth, as well as nerve function and muscle contraction.

❖ Antioxidant-Rich Berries: Mixed berries provide a rich source of antioxidants, vitamins, and minerals that help protect against oxidative stress and inflammation in the body. They're particularly high in vitamin C, which supports immune function and collagen production.

❖ Healthy Fats: Nuts are a source of healthy fats, particularly monounsaturated and polyunsaturated fats, which are beneficial for heart health and may help lower cholesterol levels.

❖ Fiber-Filled: Berries and nuts are both high in dietary fiber, which promotes digestive health, regulates blood sugar levels, and helps you feel full and satisfied. A diet rich in fiber may also help reduce the risk of chronic diseases such as heart disease, diabetes, and certain cancers.

Frozen Yogurt Bark with Berries and Nuts is a delicious and nutritious treat that's perfect for cooling off on a hot day or satisfying your sweet tooth without the guilt. With its creamy yogurt base, vibrant berries, and crunchy nuts, it's sure to be a hit with both kids and adults alike. Enjoy it as a refreshing snack or dessert any time you're craving something sweet and satisfying!

Peanut Butter Banana Ice Cream

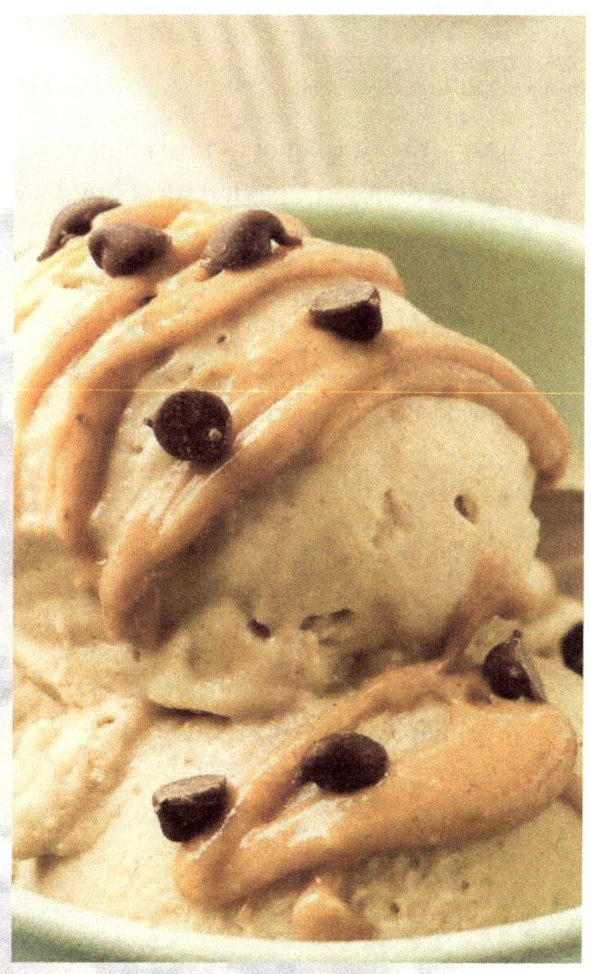

❖ **Preparation Time:** 5 minutes
❖ **Freezing Time:** 2-3 hours
❖ **Serving Unit:** Makes about 4 servings

Ingredients:

❖ 4 ripe bananas, peeled and sliced
❖ ¼ cup creamy peanut butter (or any nut or seed butter of your choice)
❖ 2 tablespoons honey or maple syrup (optional)
❖ 1 teaspoon vanilla extract
❖ Pinch of salt

❖ **Optional toppings:** chopped peanuts, chocolate chips, sliced bananas

Procedures:

Prepare the Bananas:

❖ Slice the ripe bananas into coins and place them on a baking sheet lined with parchment paper or a silicone mat.
❖ Arrange the banana slices in a single layer and freeze them for at least 2-3 hours, or until firm.

Blend the Ingredients:

❖ Once the banana slices are frozen, transfer them to a blender or food processor.
❖ Add the creamy peanut butter, honey or maple syrup (if using), vanilla extract, and a pinch of salt to the blender or food processor with the frozen banana slices.

Blend Until Smooth:

❖ Blend the mixture on high speed until smooth and creamy, scraping down the sides of the blender or food processor as needed to ensure everything is well combined.
❖ If the mixture seems too thick, you can add a splash of milk or water to help loosen it up.

Serve Immediately or Freeze:

❖ Once the peanut butter banana ice cream is smooth and creamy, you can serve it immediately for a soft-serve texture.
❖ Alternatively, you can transfer the ice cream to a container and freeze it for an additional 30 minutes to 1 hour for a firmer texture.

Garnish and Enjoy:

❖ Serve the peanut butter banana ice cream in bowls or cones.
❖ Garnish each serving with optional toppings such as chopped peanuts, chocolate chips, or sliced bananas, if desired.
❖ Enjoy the creamy and indulgent flavor of homemade peanut butter banana ice cream!

Nutritional Value (per serving):

❖ Calories: 180 kcal
❖ Protein: 4g
❖ Fat: 8g
❖ Carbohydrates: 25g
❖ Fiber: 3g
❖ Sugar: 14g

Cooking Tips:

❖ Use ripe bananas for the best flavor and sweetness. Ripe bananas will blend more easily and result in a creamier texture.
❖ If you prefer a sweeter ice cream, you can add honey or maple syrup to the mixture. However, ripe bananas provide natural sweetness, so you may not need to add any additional sweeteners.

❖ Customize the ice cream with your favorite add-ins. Chocolate chips, chopped peanuts, shredded coconut, or a drizzle of chocolate sauce are all delicious options for enhancing the flavor and texture of the ice cream.

❖ For a smoother texture, you can peel the bananas before freezing them. However, freezing the banana slices with the peel on is more convenient and helps prevent them from sticking together.

❖ If you don't have a high-powered blender or food processor, you can use a hand mixer or immersion blender to blend the ingredients. Just make sure to blend until smooth and creamy.

Health Benefits:

❖ **Naturally Sweetened:** Ripe bananas provide natural sweetness without the need for added sugars, making this ice cream a healthier alternative to store-bought varieties that are high in refined sugars.

❖ **Rich in Potassium:** Bananas are a good source of potassium, an essential mineral that helps regulate blood pressure, maintain fluid balance, and support muscle and nerve function.

❖ **Protein-Packed:** Peanut butter is rich in protein, which helps support muscle repair and growth, as well as overall health and vitality.

❖ **Healthy Fats:** Peanut butter provides heart-healthy monounsaturated fats, which may help lower cholesterol levels and reduce the risk of heart disease when consumed as part of a balanced diet.

❖ **Fiber-Filled:** Bananas and peanut butter are both high in dietary fiber, which promotes digestive health, regulates blood sugar levels, and helps you feel full and satisfied. A diet rich in fiber may also help reduce the risk of chronic diseases such as heart disease, diabetes, and certain cancers.

Peanut Butter Banana Ice Cream is a delicious and nutritious treat that's perfect for satisfying your sweet tooth while still nourishing your body with wholesome ingredients. With its creamy texture and indulgent flavor, it's sure to become a favorite dessert option for the whole family. Enjoy it as a refreshing snack on a hot day or as a guilt-free dessert any time you're craving something sweet and satisfying!

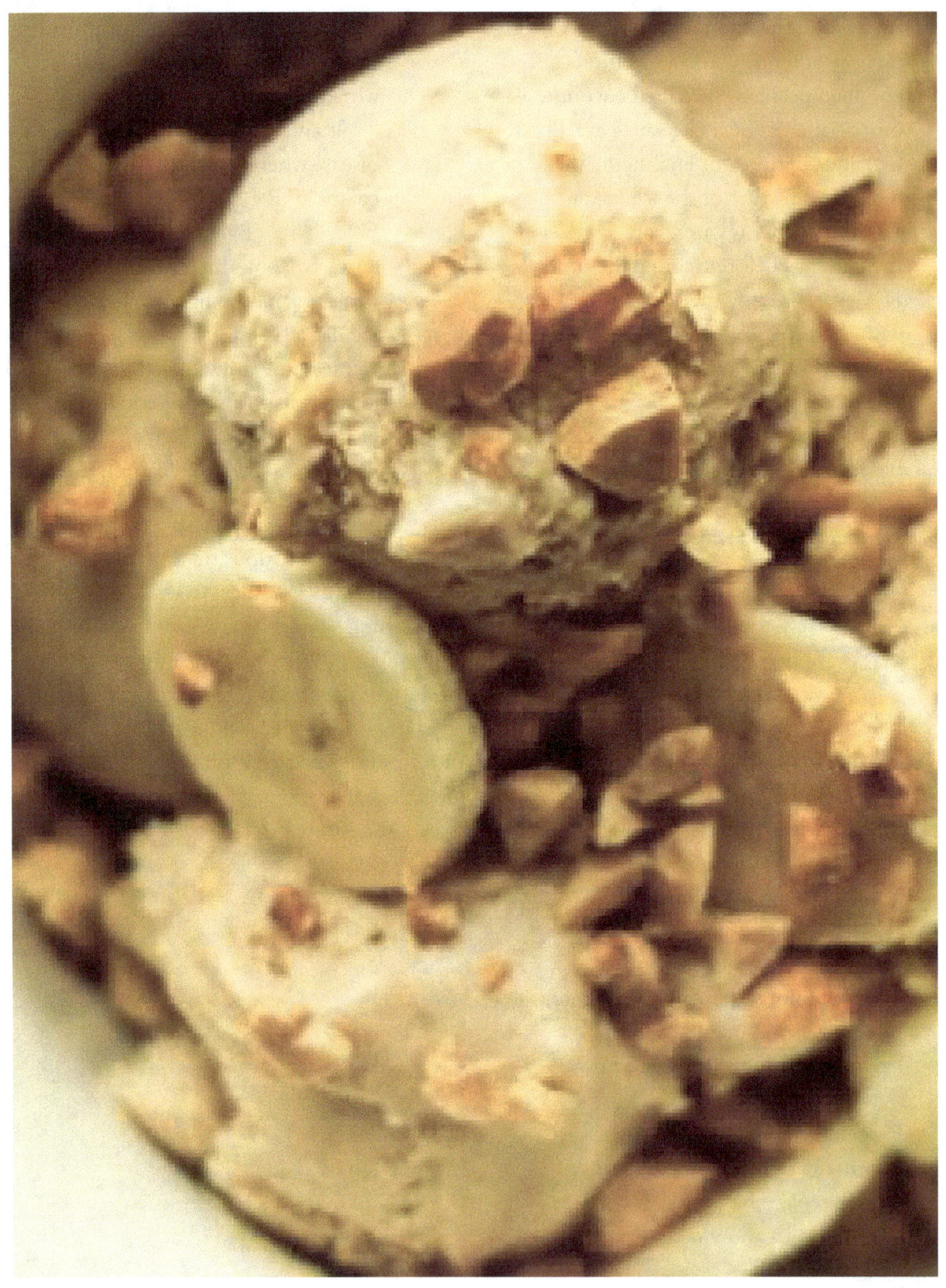

CONCLUSION

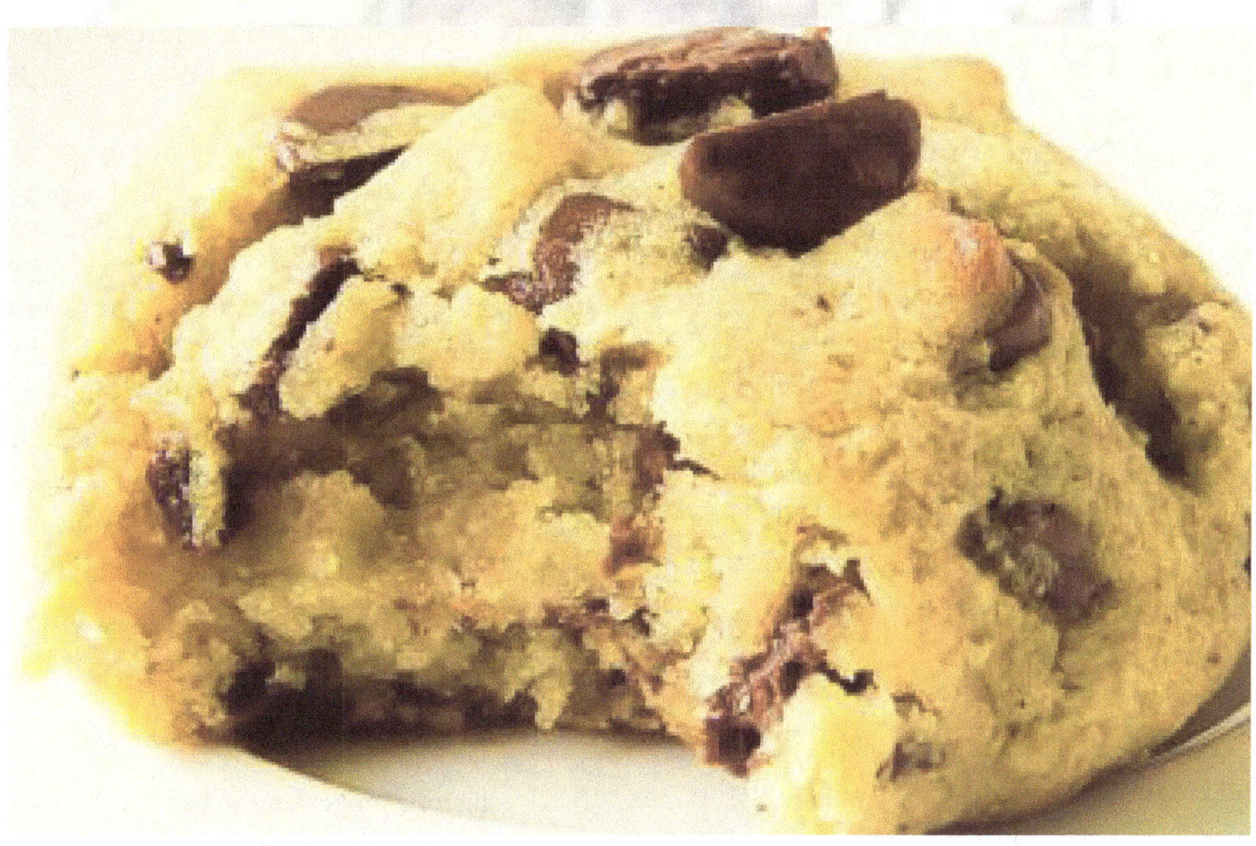

Embracing a Healthy Lifestyle with the Galveston Diet

The Galveston Diet isn't just a temporary fix or a quick weight loss solution; it's a lifestyle change that promotes long-term health and wellness. By focusing on nourishing your body with wholesome, nutrient-dense foods and incorporating regular physical activity into your daily routine, you can achieve sustainable results and improve your overall quality of life.

Final Thoughts and Encouragement

As you embark on your journey to better health and well-being with the Galveston Diet, it's important to remember that progress takes time and patience. Rome wasn't built in a day, and neither is a healthier lifestyle. Celebrate every small victory along the way, whether it's choosing a nutritious meal over processed junk food or completing a challenging workout. Each positive choice you make brings you one step closer to your goals.

It's also essential to practice self-compassion and kindness towards yourself throughout this journey. There will be times when you stumble or veer off course, and that's okay. What matters most is how you pick yourself back up and keep moving forward. Be gentle with yourself, and remember that every setback is an opportunity for growth and learning.

Share Your Experience: Testimonials and Feedback

One of the most inspiring aspects of the Galveston Diet is hearing the success stories and experiences of others who have embraced this lifestyle and transformed their health and well-being. Whether you've just started your journey or have been following the Galveston Diet for a while, sharing your story can inspire and motivate others to take control of their health and make positive changes in their lives.

If you've experienced positive results with the Galveston Diet, we encourage you to share your testimonials and feedback with the community. Your story could inspire someone who's struggling to make healthier choices or looking for support and encouragement on their own journey. Together, we can create a supportive and empowering community dedicated to living our healthiest, happiest lives.

In conclusion, embracing a healthy lifestyle with the Galveston Diet is not just about losing weight or fitting into a smaller size; it's about nourishing your body, mind, and soul with the nutrients and care it deserves. By making conscious choices to prioritize your health and well-being every day, you can create a life filled with vitality, energy, and joy. So keep pushing forward, stay committed to your goals, and remember that you have the power to create the life you desire. Here, to your health and happiness!

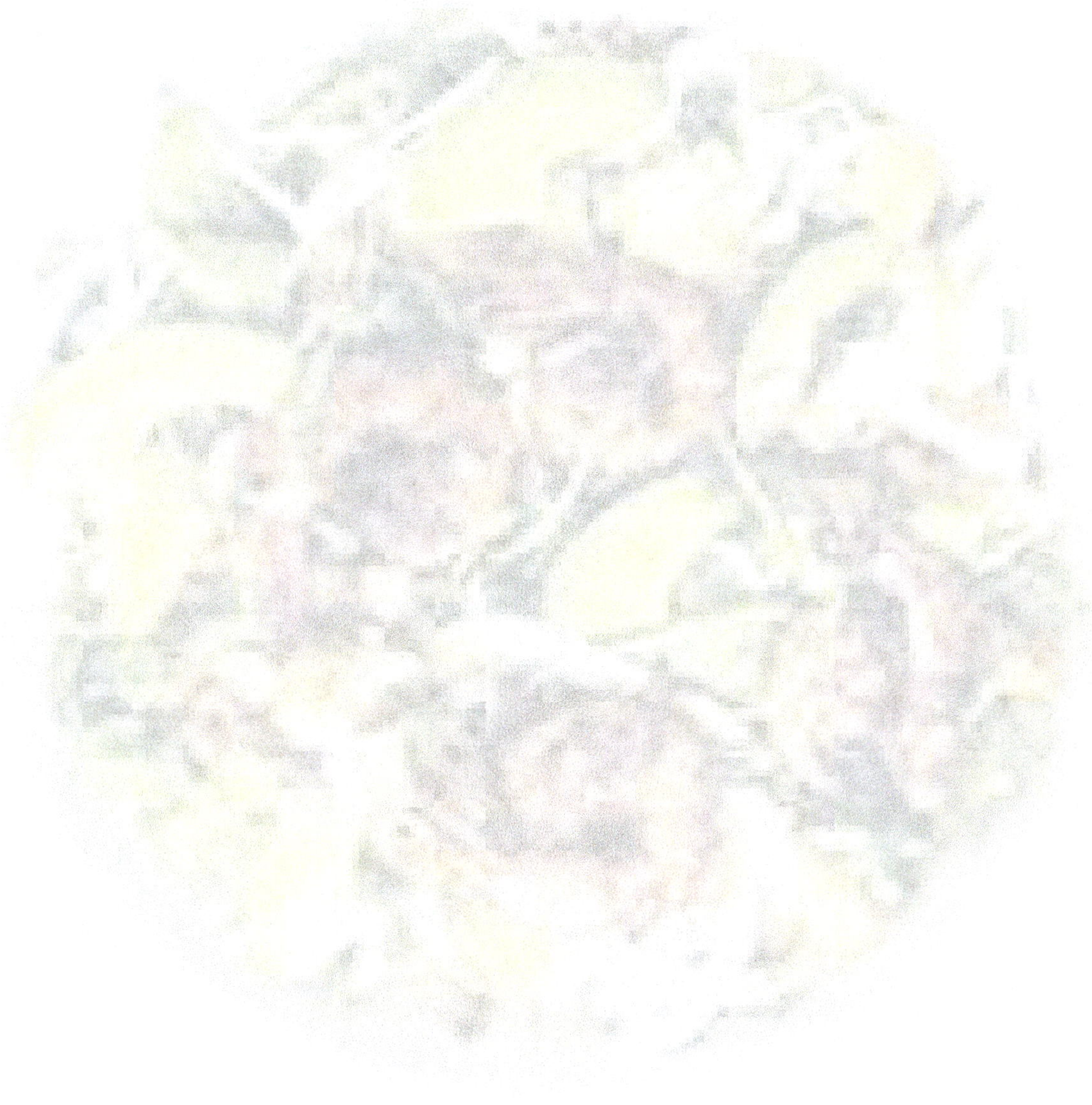

9 798328 564069